THE
FINANCIALLY
COMPETITIVE
HEALTHCARE
ORGANIZATION

The Executive's Guide
to Strategic Financial Planning
and Management

**KENNETH KAUFMAN
AND MARK HALL**

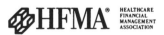

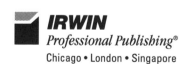

Chicago • London • Singapore

ISBN 1-55738-606-4

Printed in the United States of America

BB

BH/BJS

5 6 7 8 9 0

Dedication

To my wife, Barbara, and to my daughters, Rebecca and Sara. All of my professional efforts, including this book, have benefited immeasurably from their constant love and support.

K.K.

To my children, Brandon, Megan and Caitlin, who are both a constant source of energy and an ongoing reminder to do things right, and to my wife, Shelley, in anticipation of our life together.

M.L.H.

Contents

Acknowledgements

Some things in life are easy and some are hard. Researching and writing a book is one of the hard things. A project of this magnitude cannot be successfully completed without the help and cooperation of many people. First, we would like to thank our colleagues at Kaufman, Hall & Associates. Kaufman, Hall & Associates is not only a marvelous consulting firm but, more importantly, it is an exceptional learning environment. All of our colleagues, including Robert Carroll, Jody Hill-Mischel and Ellen Riley, have made a positive contribution to this book. Special thanks to Therese Wareham, Jason Sussman and Catherine Kleinmuntz for their contributions to Chapters 4, 5 and 6. Also our sincerest thanks to Sharon Arneson and J.D. Williams who prepared the manuscript for publication.

Ron Mills provided able and valuable editorial assistance. Mark Newton of Highland Park Hospital, Highland Park, Illinois, provided considerable insight into the difficult issues raised in Chapter 6.

The book benefited from the professional assistance provided by the staff of Probus Publishing. Our thanks to Kristine Rynne and Kevin Thornton. Kathleen Louden provided editorial assistance and the book was greatly improved by her efforts.

Finally, as we did in our last book, we would like to thank our clients. Healthcare is one of the most dynamic and fast paced industries in the American economy. Many of our clients have a financial management style that is technically expert, innovative and creative. We learn something from each client and from every engagement. Many of the best ideas in this book resulted from the day-to-day challenges of our consulting practice.

Introduction

We have written this book to help healthcare executives improve the quality of their decisionmaking. The focus of the book is on becoming and staying financially competitive.

It may be our imaginations, but recently there seems to be an increased level of interest in what constitutes excellent financial performance and how it might be achieved. As finance professionals, we are appreciative of this attention, but we also recognize that at mission-driven organizations excellent financial performance is but a means to an end. Viewed broadly over time, your organization's financial statements are nothing more than a numerical summary of the decisions made and actions taken as the organization has responded to its operating environment. Consistently excellent financial performance is helpful for three specific reasons:

1. It provides the flexibility to focus on the long view. It is hard to pay attention to anything else when the organization is experiencing financial difficulty. This is a significant problem in a changing environment. It is impossible to steer a

boat when it is listing hard to the starboard. Similarly, competitive progress depends upon establishing and maintaining financial equilibrium.

2. It increases organizational self esteem. Everyone likes to play for a winning team. Financial performance is a critical and easily understood element of the scorecard. Financially competitive organizations are unlikely to experience the "under-siege" mentality which is so common in the industry today. Steady, measurable progress towards well understood goals is the key to success. The alternative to financial self esteem is the upsize-downsize cycle which is so destructive to an organization's spirit.

3. The capital markets demand it. Access to affordable capital is essential for long-term survival. Spotty, inconsistent performance compromises that access. This will be particularly true as the industry completes its transition from the regulated model to the competitive/reform model.

It is ironic that, as the industry focus has become increasingly dominated by financial concerns, the finance staff is increasingly unable to do anything to improve financial performance through its direct intervention. The decisions that are made day in and day out in the operating departments and on the nursing floors are the primary drivers of financial performance. Excellent financial performance is, therefore, primarily the responsibility of the non-financial managers of the organization, both at the executive and at the department level. Unfortunately, many of these individuals are operating without a sense of financial vision or an understanding of how their individual decisions affect the whole. As one laboratory director put it to us after a presentation on her hospital's long-term financial plan, "If I'd known about this two weeks ago, I'd have done a lot of things differently." It is our belief that this comment reflects a common situation. We are confident that, given adequate analysis and communication, there is sufficient capability throughout the organization to understand and respond to these issues. If we are wrong on this, the future will be most unpleasant.

The book is organized around the attitudes, tools and processes which must be in place for your organization to make good financial decisions. Its emphasis is on the systematic application of corporate finance principles. It is meant for financial and non-financial executives who wish to be more effective producers and consumers of financial data and analysis. The first three chapters provide a theoretical foundation; we have tried, where appropriate, to use case studies to make our points clear. The last three chapters were developed to reinforce the concepts described in the first half of the book and apply them in an in-depth fashion to specific situations. Each chapter is meant to stand on its own, but the book is best understood if the chapters are taken in sequence.

Chapter 1, *Executive Decisionmaking in Healthcare: A Financial Planning Perspective,* examines the reasons why decisionmaking has become so difficult lately and considers the applicability of both intuition and

analysis to the management problem. It concludes
with a discussion of the ten attributes of financially
competitive healthcare organizations.

To be effective, your organization needs to understand where it is financially, where it needs to go and
what critical variables must be managed to get there.
Chapter 2, *Financial Planning for Competitive Performance*, describes a process for developing a strategic financial plan and for communicating that plan to your
organization. Credit analysis, financial ratios, debt capacity and the reasoned setting of financial goals are
some of the specific topics considered.

Effective financial planning helps to create capital
capacity for the financially competitive healthcare
provider. Wise use of this capital requires well-devel-
oped capital deployment skills. These skills are the
subject of Chapter 3, *Capital Deployment, Corporate Finance and Constructive Decisionmaking*. The chapter focuses on the incremental analysis of individual initiatives, with particular attention paid to net present
value analysis and an approach for allocating capital
among competing uses.

As the industry consolidates, the remaining players
will have the opportunity to evaluate numerous acquisition opportunities. The ability to distinguish between the good, the bad and the ugly and to determine acquisition prices which represent good uses of
scarce capital will be important survival skills. Chapter 4, *Analysis of Acquisitions*, applies the material presented in Chapter 3 to the special case of acquisition
through the examination of three case studies. The
chapter emphasizes the quantitative techniques em-

ployed and describes how these techniques were used to support actual negotiations.

At some point in its life cycle, every healthcare organization is faced with a project expenditure which has the potential to fundamentally alter its capital, financial and competitive position. In many cases, implementation of the project will require a commitment to reposition the organization financially and operationally. Chapter 5, *Analysis and Sizing of Project Investments*, is a case study in how the strategic financial planning concepts elucidated in Chapter 2 may be used to bring financial order to the consideration of a major infrastructure project.

Physician-hospital integration activities are a significant concern in today's evolving healthcare environment. Our point in Chapter 6, *Physician-Hospital Integration Analysis*, is that the quality of the financial analysis which is brought to bear on these efforts can have a significant effect on their success. The chapter lays out a five-step process which we have found to be applicable to nearly all situations and applies that process to an actual case.

The Afterword, *Quantitative Reasoning and the Financially Competitive Healthcare Organization*, brings us back to where we started. It applies some general observations made by others about the fallibility of human reasoning to the current state of healthcare organizations and delineates the role that financial leadership and careful quantitative analysis can play in helping to assure that your organization lives up to its potential.

Much attention is currently focused on what's wrong with the healthcare industry and the woes it will face in the future. Frankly, we're hard pressed to identify a historical period of the industry more interesting and challenging than the present. The changes that are taking place offer the potential for the accomplishment of many worthwhile objectives. The good news is that the available information base and the decision support technology is increasingly up to the challenge. The success of your organization will in large measure be a result of its willingness and ability to employ the available tools.

CHAPTER 1

Kenneth Kaufman

Executive Decisionmaking in Healthcare: A Financial Planning Perspective

Decisionmaking in healthcare organizations for years has been seen as a fine art guided by the hard lessons of trial and error. Healthcare executives, who have a just pride in their craft and tenacity, have been much less comfortable with quantitative analysis than have their corporate counterparts and instead have preferred to rely on experience and intuition to guide their decisionmaking.

Now, however, healthcare organizations, like so many other organizations, are finding even simple decisions difficult to make. The causes of this decision-making distress, as identified by Efraim Turban, noted professor of computer science, can be traced to three areas of change:

1. *Burgeoning technologies and improved communications,* which present an ever-widening selection of alternatives.

2. *Greater uncertainty* in the healthcare industry, which makes it difficult to predict the consequences of any decision.

3. *The higher cost of making an error,* given the complexity and magnitude of operations, swift automation, and the chain reaction an error may cause in many parts of the contemporary organization.

No healthcare executive today can survive by wits alone, and no healthcare organization can flourish with data that are poor or poorly interpreted. Sound financial planning begins with a thorough understanding of organizational decisionmaking and executive judgment.

Managing with Both Sides of the Brain

Organizational decisions, as assessed by Herbert Simon, fall into two broad categories: structured and unstructured. Structured decisions are repetitive, dealing with routine matters. Unstructured decisions are new or uncommon requiring sometimes creative solutions to complex problems. Most of the important decisions that a healthcare organization faces are unstructured. Plotting managed care strategy; configuring efficient staffing relationships; electing appropriate clinical programs; deftly assessing acquisition, divestiture, and network activities—such complex endeavors call for unstructured decisions.

Both structured and unstructured decisions demand structured thinking. Luckily, an executive's brain has two lobes: one to behold or admire the complexity and novelty of a situation and one to formulate a workable resolution. Some would call it management by intuition, but even intuition, Harry Davis and Robin Hogarth, professors at the University of Chicago, argue, is learned largely from experience. How well one learns the lessons of experience, though, depends on how insightfully one lives the experience and how faithfully one interprets it. "Mere activity," as John Dewey observed, "does not constitute experience." Every musician or athlete knows the difference between practice and *good* practice, and consistent performers have an uncanny ability to make every practice session a good one. The capable executive likewise knows the difference between dependable feedback and ambiguous feedback. Dependable feedback informs what we later perceive to be good intuition, whereas ambiguous feedback leaves the decisionmaker stumbling in the dark.

The message should be plain: intuition alone is a highly unreliable executive tool. The truly insightful executive confronts the organization's unstructured decisions with a ready store of technically supportive and conceptually accurate data. To compete in today's economic environment, healthcare organizations must give their executives the information they need to develop their decisionmaking skills. The most reliable feedback is the result of highly quantitative and highly structured analytic techniques.

The Financially Capable Healthcare Organization

In our experience, the constructive use of analytic techniques and decision-support tools is the hallmark of what we call the financially capable healthcare organization. Such organizations embrace principles and values that promote decisionmaking processes that are rational, consistent, quantitative, and, most important, competent. They value skepticism and experimentation and choose reliable data and rigorous analysis over the favored political solution of the moment. In short, the financially capable organization employs a decisionmaking philosophy born of and borne by scientific methods.

But what are the distinguishing characteristics of healthcare organizations that consistently achieve excellent financial and organizational performance? What attitudes and values must be in place to create a decisionmaking process that can harness an organization's collective good judgment?

The financially capable healthcare organization has ten key attributes listed below.

1. *The chief executive officer has conceived a financial vision.* Show us a successful healthcare organization, and we'll show you a CEO who sets concrete financial goals and objectives and clearly articulates them to the board and management

team. So essential is this component of executive leadership that, in our experience, it cannot be delegated. No one but the CEO can set the financial vision for the organization.

But CEOs are often reluctant financial leaders. For too long, too many healthcare CEOs have been attempting to manage financially complex organizations without the requisite financial tools and skills. Because many healthcare CEOs lack formal financial training or experience, they are often uncomfortable with the responsibility of setting a long-term financial direction for the organization.

Although chief financial officers can and often do provide leadership in this critical area, executing the financial vision requires the active participation of the entire organization, including divisions and individuals over whom the CFO may exercise little control or influence. Reaching certain financial goals may require, for example, significant expense cuts or implementation of radically different patterns of medical staff practice. Only the chief executive has the authority and span of control to direct such diverse changes in the organization's day-to-day management.

Time and again we have watched organizations set out on a particular financial course, only to lose their way at the first sign of trouble. Most often, the CEO either didn't understand the strategic financial direction or never completely committed to it. The CEO's involvement in setting financial goals and objectives is a pre-requisite to an organization's financial success. Issues of vision and leadership are a critical part of the CEO's job description, and vision and leadership are necessary elements that support an organization's long-term financial performance.

2. *Management follows the simple rule, "What gets measured, gets done."* Major commercial organizations measure every aspect of their operations because they believe the old tenet, "What gets measured gets done." Financially capable healthcare organizations do the same. They measure inputs and outcomes, compare them to established norms, and provide regular feedback to their managers.

   Financially astute healthcare executives are not lost in a thicket of data. They know, for example, that in their hospital a census of 280 inpatients and 1,000 outpatient visits per day with an overall case mix index of 1.5 implies a staffing ratio of 4.2 full-time equivalent employees (FTEs) per adjusted occupied bed. If, for a month under these conditions, staffing increases to 4.4 FTEs per adjusted occupied bed, the capable executive knows how to identify the cause and quickly bring the staffing ratio back to equilibrium.

   For many years, healthcare managers thought that the process of delivering care was too complex for traditional production line measurement. Now, with pressure from all manner of external constituencies and the advent of superior data collection techniques, all types of inputs and outcomes are easily measured and reported.

3. *Management understands and applies principles of corporate finance.* Consider again the difficulty of financial decisionmaking in healthcare today, and the high cost of mistakes in an environment of such complexity and uncertainty. How do financially capable organizations cope? They begin by building upon the strongest of foundations: the principles of corporate finance.

The capable organization seeks order. Order in this case can be defined as the use of consistent techniques to analyze and evaluate complex business problems. The principles of corporate finance impose mathematical order over essentially chaotic decisionmaking. A net present value analysis, for example, distills all of an investment's characteristics down to a simple dollar value, enabling the organization to evaluate the investment on its own merits or to properly compare it with other investment opportunities.

Remember: every decision an organization makes either adds to or reduces the value of the overall operation. The cumulative effect of these incremental decisions determines the organization's future financial success. Application of the principles of corporate finance enables the organization to measure the impact of each decision.

Given a technically capable finance department, senior management can aggressively incorporate analyses into the decisionmaking process, and the board (or other governing body) can depend on the numbers to validate the organization's key strategic moves.

4. *Management has a sophisticated financial plan.* The financial plan is the backbone of the financially capable healthcare organization. Not to be confused with the budget, which is the annual plan that allocates human and capital resources, the financial plan quantitatively evaluates the organization's financial risk given alternative scenarios. The sophisticated financial plan identifies corrective actions that the organization can make in response to certain expected or unexpected changes.

   In business, as in sports, the team that best executes its plan is usually the winner. A sophisticated financial planning process enables the capable healthcare organization to execute. Logical and informed financial decisions give an organization the competitive edge in a marketplace whose changing needs demand quick response. Internally, a good financial plan lends the overall strategic plan a sharper focus and stronger momentum by bridging the gap between strategies and actions.

5. *The organization favors a quantitative capital allocation process.* Providing state-of-the-art healthcare is a capital-intensive proposition, and healthcare organizations' overall requirements for capital may increase as the industry continues to con-

solidate. Despite the importance of such decisions and the fact that capital is a scarce resource, many organizations select their capital investments haphazardly, valuing political input over rigorous analysis.

Capital allocation is a process that requires the rigorous and consistent application of proven quantitative techniques. Financial planning, financial statement projections, project analysis, and present value analysis all contribute to the evaluation of capital investments and dramatically increase the probability of selecting investments that will increase the long-term value of the organization.

As a general rule, poorly managed organizations consistently make poor investment decisions. Although the danger signs of poor short-term financial management—operating losses, inadequate cash flow, an inability to collect receivables promptly—are readily apparent, inappropriate capital allocations take more time to reveal themselves. However, an imprudent capital investment can gradually erode the financial integrity of the organization.

6. *Management consistently applies quantitative decision-support tools.* The financially capable organization distrusts intuitive solutions to complex business problems. This does not mean that the capable organization is afraid to make intuitive decisions but that it prefers to give its decision-making team a sound analytical footing on which to work. The executive team is comfort-

able with a wide variety of decision-support tools and is able to routinely prepare detailed financial projections for the organization as a whole and for the specific problem at hand.

The financially capable organization also employs a highly integrated planning process that instantly can show the financial impacts of changes to the strategic plan. This real-time decision-support structure allows for immediate analysis, consistent and reliable feedback, and improved communication, all prerequisites for first-class financial decisionmaking in our turbulent healthcare environment.

7. *Management sets annual financial goals and objectives, welcoming organizationwide input.* All successful organizations set firm, measurable goals and objectives. And every member of the organization, given the opportunity and enough information, can participate in achieving those goals and objectives. The financially capable organization makes its financial goals and objectives known and understood among its key constituencies—management, the board, medical staff, the community, and the capital markets. By doing so, it cultivates an organizationwide sense of ownership in its financial direction.

Instead of simply declaring that it will strive, for example, to better its cash position from $25 million to $50 million, the financially capable organization explains why and how. The organization's ultimate objective in setting such a goal might be to increase its bond rating from

"A-" to "A." Financial leaders should present the goal, reveal its underlying objective, and perhaps supply a supporting credit analysis in a carefully prepared package that all can understand. Briefed with such easy-to-follow materials, the key constituencies can actively participate in setting the financial goals and objectives that, after all, cannot be achieved without their aid and cooperation.

8. *The organization has a visible operating plan and disseminates its financial goals.* An indispensable corollary to the rule "what gets measured, gets done" is the sociological theorem "visibility of consequences"; if you want to encourage or discourage certain behavior within your organization, you must make the consequences of such behavior highly visible. This is especially true for behavior that influences the financial performance of a healthcare provider.

A financial plan quantitatively defines the profitability and liquidity requirements of the organization. Meeting those requirements requires setting objectives and goals. But the successful organization goes a step further, organizing its financial goals and objectives into an operating plan and giving that operating plan wide visibility within the organization. Once the results of the operating plan have been measured, those results also are given wide visibility.

This internal benchmarking process allows the organization to make quick and necessary adjustments to the operating plan so that it can meet the goals and objectives of the financial plan.

9. *The organization has a strategic plan that takes into account the requirements of the capital markets.* Financially capable organizations understand that the most important factor in their continued financial and strategic success is ready access to capital at a competitive cost. The competent healthcare organization has a high capital markets IQ. Issues such as access to bond insurance or how to improve bond ratings are key factors in the planning process. The financially capable organization stays close to the capital markets and considers the credit community one of its key constituencies.

10. *Management reduces expenses while improving service and quality.* The healthcare environment is in a state of great flux. With the federal government in the lead, and other payers not far behind, the entire provider system and its traditional "power and influence" relationships are being turned upside down. But many organizations become completely focused on this environment; all of the important issues appear to be external. The chaos outside becomes the chaos inside.

   Financially capable organizations are not easily diverted. Their management focus is strongly biased toward issues that the organization can control or at least directly influence. As a result, the financially capable organization tends to have a heavy focus on controlling costs and expenses and an aggressive attitude toward improving service and quality.

Faced with a decrease in profitability, for example, the passive organization first looks for techniques that might increase revenue; the financially capable organization aggressively reduces costs to meet profitability goals.

Sometimes the results are the same, but the difference in attitude is material and significant to the long-term financial success of the organization.

Conclusion

Think of the decisionmaking process in algebraic terms. An appropriate formula might be:

(Intuition + Experience) (Quantitative feedback + Organized analysis) = Organizational competence

The point is that the application of intuition plus experience without the benefit of analysis is just guessing, but the use of quantitative techniques without the buffer of experience and judgment is a meaningless mathematical exercise. Sophisticated financial planning creates a necessary and consistent context for able decisionmaking, despite uncertain and complex circumstances, and permits the informed application of executive judgment.

CHAPTER 2

Kenneth Kaufman

Financial Planning for Competitive Performance

The future will be brighter for the healthcare organization that develops and executes a sound financial plan. A financial plan articulates future financial risk in quantitative terms, considers likely alternative scenarios, and specifies prudent reactions to expected or unexpected changes. The plan links the organization's strategic vision to measurable financial objectives, which permits the organization to react quickly to a dynamic marketplace. This combination of analytic rigor and ready adaptability inspires confident executive leadership and excellent decisionmaking.

Financial planning requires the full participation of both the CEO and CFO as well as the participation of managers who make the organization's decisions and

enact the organization's vision. Nowhere will the organization's ability to disseminate information, allocate resources and responsibilities, and make decisions be put to a tougher test than in the financial
planning process. A well-crafted financial plan en-
courages all employees to do their best and creates a
participatory environment in which the organization's
broader strategic planning process can thrive as well.

Of course, financial planners and decisionmakers,
including executives, board members, senior management, and medical staff leadership, must understand
the quantitative financial information they gather
and, more importantly, must be fully prepared to use
that information to achieve the organization's strategic and financial objectives. In particular, all must
have a firm grasp of the three building blocks of the
financial plan:

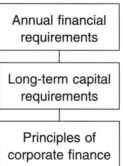

In this chapter we define an organization's annual
financial requirements and long-term capital requirements and demonstrate the application of some basic
principles of corporate finance. We also present a case
study that demonstrates the financial planning process at a midsized community hospital.

Defining Annual Financial Requirements

A journey of a thousand miles begins with a single step, as the old saying goes. So the healthcare financial plan, which looks five or more years into an uncertain future, must begin with a reliable definition of financial requirements in year one. Requirements for each following year must be just as carefully defined so that the organization can reach its longer-term goals and objectives. At bottom, the financial plan is only as sound as its weakest year.

An organization's annual financial requirements are fivefold:

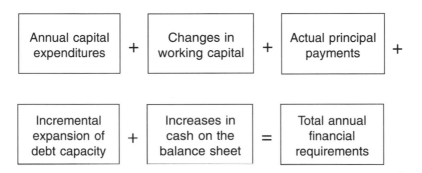

The first three requirements (planned capital expenditures to meet operating needs for the year, plus any expected changes in working capital, plus principal payments) must be met every year just to maintain subsistence-level financial performance. Competitive financial performance, on the other hand, requires the forward thinking represented by the last two items (annual expansion of debt capacity and increases in cash on the balance sheet). Debt capacity and cash reserves are the organization's seed corn.

Debt capacity describes the amount of debt the organization is capable of supporting. Every organization that intends to remain financially competitive in the long run must expand its debt capacity year by year. The capacity to incur additional debt makes the organization more responsive to its market and more resilient to expected and unexpected changes. For example, a hospital with a total debt capacity of $30 million and outstanding debt of $25 million has a net debt capacity of $5 million. If the hospital plans to renovate a wing by two years from now at a projected cost of $20 million, the financial plan should describe the incremental amount of debt capacity that must be added to the balance sheet every year to raise the extra $15 million for the project.

Increases in cash on the balance sheet must be accomplished every year because each healthcare organization needs cash (1) to respond to the changing healthcare environment and (2) to preserve its creditworthiness. Unresponsive and uncreditworthy organizations will have no place in the healthcare markets of the near future. Unless an organization has already accumulated all the cash it will need for the next five years, building up the necessary cash reserve will require a financial plan that specifies incremental and progressive annual cash goals.

Doing the Math at the Margin

Having defined the financial requirements for each year of the planning period, the organization is now ready to plot its long-term financial requirements to achieve competitive financial performance. Figure 2-1 depicts a five-year financial plan, highlighting the difference between mere financial survival and truly competitive performance. The "Survival Financial Performance" line, remember, represents the requirements for annual capital expenditures, plus working capital, plus principal payments. The area between the "Survival Financial Performance" line and the "Competitive Financial Performance" line represents the amount of cash required for the organization to be financially competitive. The slope of the "Competitive Financial Performance" line describes the organization's requirement for year-by-year increases in cash reserves and debt capacity.

Figure 2-1 Long Term Financial Requirements

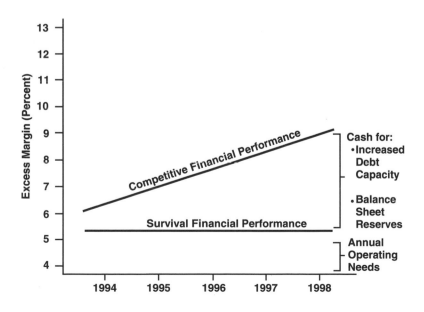

This figure provides an excellent tool for explaining to the board, medical staff, and senior management the incremental impacts of significant decisions. We call it "doing the math at the margin." Once the slope of the organization's competitive financial performance has been determined, every decision should be geared toward keeping to that slope. Any decision or initiative that runs contrary to the planned course might threaten the organization's financial ability to compete in the market over the long term. The graph enables financial planners to portray each decision as having an incrementally positive, neutral, or negative effect on the organization's long-term competitive position.

Defining Long-Term Capital Requirements

Because capital expenditures are the key variable in determining an organization's long-term financial requirements, the organization must be especially diligent in defining its current capital position and projecting its capital requirements for the planning period. Which programs are affordable? How should they be financed? How will they affect the organization overall? For executives to make such judgments, they must be able to predict the financial effects of their decisions.

Asking the Right Questions

A robust financial planning process creates a reliable means of assessing the long-term implications of every capital expenditure. Specifically, the financial planning process answers seven crucial questions:

1. What are the organization's strategic capital requirements?

2. How much cash should the organization have?

3. How much debt can the organization afford?

4. What is the magnitude of the organization's capital shortfall?

5. What short- and long-term profitability targets are necessary to resolve the shortfall?

6. What is the required level of operating change to meet the targets?

7. Where is the capital going to come from in the short and long term?

Any healthcare organization that expects to succeed in the current and future environments must place the answers to these questions at decisionmakers' fingertips.

- *What are the organization's strategic capital requirements?* The financial plan is inseparable from the strategic plan it serves. Guided by a sound strategy, the organization must determine its complete capital needs to achieve competitive financial performance. A one- or two-year financial planning horizon is too shortsighted for most healthcare organizations today; more likely, years one and two should be spent accumulating the cash and debt capacity to fund the capital projects planned for years four and five. Just as in strategic planning, financial planning begins with a long-range vision and then works backward to schedule the action steps required to fulfill that vision.

- *How much cash should the organization have? How much debt can the organization afford?* These are probably the two most important questions a healthcare organization must ask itself. Creditworthiness (discussed in the next section) and adequate access to capital are dependent on the organization's liquidity and its ability to renew its capital capacity by repaying existing debt and maintaining a bottom line that provides for necessary incremental increases in debt capacity. The specification and quantification of these two variables are critical steps in developing the algebra that is necessary to solve the financial planning equation.

- *What is the magnitude of the organization's capital shortfall?* Financial planners must measure the organization's relative capital position at frequent intervals. Capital surpluses or shortfalls are easy enough to calculate:

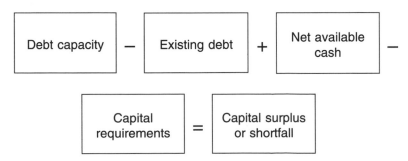

Decisionmakers cannot be expected to do the math at the margin if they don't know where the margin is. The financial plan gives accurate, up-to-date readings.

- *What short- and long-term profitability targets are necessary to resolve the shortfall?* The financial planning process identifies the relationship between profitability, debt capacity, and capital spending. It demonstrates that a specific level of capital spending is directly related to a specific level of profitability and that, if profitability targets are not met, capital spending levels must be reduced. For many line managers, these findings show for the first time that day-to-day management has a real effect on capital investment.

- *What is the required level of operating change to meet the targets?* Absent any dramatic increases in revenue, generating capital will often require a real reduction in operating expenses. Few organizations in the current environment can afford both more capital and an increase in day-to-day expenses. The financial plan provides an objective measure of the expense controls necessary to provide a given amount of capital over a specified period. The financial plan measures the depth of the required trade-off and clearly displays that information, giving the board and management team a real choice between capital investments and cuts in operating expenses.

- *Where is the capital going to come from in the short and long term?* This is the last question that planners should ask. The capital markets should not be approached until all long-term financial requirements have been identified and all the right steps have been taken to ensure the organization's financial capability to pursue its strategic plans.

Asking these straightforward questions is a discipline all organizations must practice. Generating precise input data, widely circulating that information among decisionmakers, and acting in concert to answer these questions—these are the hallmarks of the competitive healthcare organization.

Creditworthiness

Preparing and maintaining a credit analysis is the first step of the financial plan. The credit analysis allows the healthcare organization to compare its recent financial performance to relevant national standards. This type of analysis is accomplished, of course, through the use of ratio analysis. Many CFOs shy away from comparative credit analyses because they believe the analysis raises more questions than it answers. Questions include what ratios should comprise the analysis, what should be the standard of comparison, and what should be the relevant interpretations. While there are at least 50 ratios which could comprise a credit analysis, we believe that the use of eight ratios can serve as the key indicators of financial strength and weakness and provide a benchmark of past and current creditworthiness.

The eight key ratios are as follows:

- *Debt service coverage* measures the factor by which cash flow covers debt service.

- *Operating margin* reflects the profitability from operations.

- *Excess margin* defines profitability from operations plus nonoperating revenue.

- *Debt-to-capitalization ratio* indicates how highly leveraged, or debt financed, the organization is; the higher the capitalization ratio, the higher the risk.

- *Cushion ratio*—probably the most important credit ratio in use today—compares the organization's free cash to its annual debt service.

- *Days cash on hand*, another gauge of liquidity, tells how many days of cash operating expenses the organization has set aside.

- *Average days in accounts receivable* measures the timeliness of collections and is widely considered to be an accurate barometer of financial management.

- *Average age of plant* measures the age of physical facilities and technology and puts the other ratios into perspective by answering the question, How pressing is the organization's need for capital?

The definitions of the above ratios are provided in Table 2-1.

Table 2-1 Definitions of Financial Ratios

Debt service coverage:

$$\frac{(\text{Excess revenue over expenses} + \text{Depreciation} + \text{Interest} + \text{Amortization})}{\text{Annual debt service}}$$

Operating margin:

$$\frac{\text{Total operating revenue} - \text{Operating expenses}}{\text{Total operating revenue}}$$

Excess margin:

$$\frac{\text{Income from operations} + \text{Nonoperating revenue}}{\text{Total operating} + \text{Nonoperating revenue}}$$

Capitalization ratio:

$$\frac{\text{Long}-\text{term debt (less current portion)}}{\text{Long}-\text{term debt (less current portion)} + \text{Fund balance}}$$

Average days in accounts receivable (net):

$$\left(\frac{\text{Accounts receivable net of reserves}}{\text{Net patient revenue less bad debt expense}}\right) \times 365$$

Cushion ratio:

$$\frac{\text{Cash and marketable securities} + \text{Board designated funds}}{\text{Annual debt service}}$$

Days cash on hand:

$$\frac{(\text{Cash and marketable securities} + \text{Board designated funds})}{\text{Total operating expenses} - \text{Depreciation}} \times 365$$

Average age of plant:

$$\text{Accumulated depreciation} / \text{Depreciation expense}$$

Performing the Right Analyses

The best financial performers are sophisticated inter-
preters of essential financial data. Most healthcare organizations today employ automated modeling software and techniques to help them gather, process, and
circulate vital financial information. Computer mod-

els allow planners to test the financial impact of decisions before the organization commits to a long-term strategy.

To be successful, your financial model must integrate eight steps into the organization's permanent financial planning process:

1. Produce *high-quality financial projections* that decisionmakers will find reliable and that will withstand the scrutiny of the investment community.

2. Perform *macroanalyses* and *financial goal setting* to help plot the organization's long-term strategies.

3. Perform *microanalyses* and *project evaluations* to assess individual capital investment opportunities.

4. Creatively use *sensitivity and target analyses* to adjust the model for a number of scenarios, such as changes in reimbursement, declining utilization, or increases in overall costs.

5. Develop *five-year capital expenditure estimates* to establish the organization's slope of competitive financial performance.

6. Perform *real-time debt capacity analysis* to determine in an instant what changes are necessary to meet future debt capacity requirements.

7. Establish the organization's *financial and capital position* to define the capital shortfall that must be overcome.

8. Calculate *the relationship between operating profit-ability and given levels of capital expenditures* to show how well the organization must perform to pursue its capital investment goals.

Performing excellent analyses is not enough, of course. The challenge is to put this information to good use. So the model must go a step further, inte-grating steps 1 through 8 into a visible operating plan that defines the specific actions that must be taken to meet the organization's financial goals and objectives.

The best way to explain how the financial, strategic, and operating plans can work together is by examin-ing a practical case study.

A Case Study: Financial Planning

Community Medical Center, a 250-bed hospital lo-cated in a midsized city, faces decreasing occupancy rates of inpatient beds and a static population in its service area. It competes with the other medical center across town, creating an overbedded market that threatens the financial future of both hospitals. Al-though historical operations have been generally ac-ceptable, Community Medical Center's leaders are concerned about the organization's continuing ability to invest in its future. Specifically, they are fearful that the medical center may lose out in a potential merger unless they can improve its financial position.

The first order of business is to define the financial and capital requirements necessary to assure the or-ganization's creditworthiness. Community Medical Center has to answer some tough questions:

- What level of long-term capital investment is required to maintain competitive facilities?

- What level of annual financial performance is necessary to fund the required capital investment?

- Given the calculated level of appropriate financial performance, can that level of performance realistically be achieved?

- Is the organization comfortable with the level of risk required by the operating plan?

These questions can best be answered through a series of comparative analyses, beginning with a look at how Community Medical Center's financial results stack up against national credit averages. These analyses will generate all the information the medical center requires to define its long-term financial requirements and to establish an operating plan to meet those requirements.

In short, the following analyses constitute Community Medical Center's financial plan.

Is Community Medical Center Creditworthy?

It may seem odd to worry about national data when the competition in town poses a real and immediate threat. However, that is the discipline of financial planning. Remember that Community Medical Center is competing for capital in a national marketplace. A healthcare organization's long-term competitive position is substantially dependent on its ability to raise affordable capital in the debt markets. The financial plan is a calculus that revolves around the definition of a series of constraints and the identification of a series of key variables. The first constraint that creates the basis for the financial plan is the hospital's bond rating. The board and management must either maintain or attain a minimum bond rating that permits the medical center to effectively compete in its local marketplace.

The credit analysis for Community Medical Center is summarized in Table 2-2.

What are the key observations that can be made from the results provided in Table 2-2? First, the profitability ratios (debt service coverage, operating margin, and excess margin) are, for the most part, close to national medians for hospitals rated "A–." The trend, however, is distinctly negative.

For example, the hospital's excess margin in 1991 was a reasonable 4.5%, but by 1993 had deteriorated to 2.6 percent. The debt-to-capitalization ratio measures total leverage. The current capitalization ratio at the hospital is 50.3 percent. The trend is downward and in the right direction but the ratio of 50.3 percent is still significantly above the "A–" national median of 41.4 percent.

The cushion ratio and the days cash on hand ratio measure liquidity. Liquidity is probably the single most important measure of creditworthiness in the current capital markets environment. Note in Table 2-2 that the "A–" medians in 1992 were 4.6x and 104 days, for cushion ratio and days cash on hand, respec-

Table 2-2   Credit Analysis for Medical Center

Ratio	S & P "A–" Rated Medical Centers[a]	Medical Center		
		1991	1992	1993
Debt Service Coverage	2.4x	2.0x	1.9x	2.2x
Operating Margin	3.45%	4.2%	2.8%	2.2%
Excess Margin	5.46%	4.5%	3.6%	2.6%
Debt/Capitalization	41.4%	54.7%	50.8%	50.3%
Cushion Ratio	4.66x	.38x	.11x	.49x
Days Cash on Hand	104.1 days	13.6 days	6.5 days	12.7 days
Days in Accounts Receivable (Net)	66.2 days	71.1 days	80.9 days	84.6 days
Average Age of Plant		6.5 years	7.2 years	7.1 years

[a] Reflects Standard & Poor's medians for medical centers rated "A–" in 1992.

tively. This part of the analysis tells the real story: Community Medical Center effectively has no cash.

The final key ratio is the average age of plant. The average age of plant, when looked at by itself, is not always instructive. When evaluated in combination with the liquidity ratios and the leverage ratios, it can provide unique insights. In this case, the hospital's leverage ratio is relatively high while the cash position is quite low. Under these circumstances, we would expect that much of the money spent, both debt and cash, would have been invested in physical plant and that this investment would be reflected by a low average age of plant ratio. Indeed, in our example, this does prove to be the case.

Our conclusions from all of the above are important. First, the overall financial condition of Community Medical Center is deteriorating and that deterioration is significant. Second, the hospital no longer has an "A–" credit and, if it attempted to raise money in the debt markets on the merits of its current financial performance, it most likely would receive a "BBB" category credit rating. This analysis sets the stage for the remainder of the financial plan and assists in creating a framework for the development of long-term financial goals and targets.

Is the Medical Center Spending Too Much or Too Little for Capital?

How much should we be investing? This simple question is a source of endless confusion for many hospital boards.

Table 2-3   Estimate of Total Capital Requirements

	1993	1994	1995	1996	1997	1998	1994-98 Total
Identified Capital ($000s)		$13,672	$12,872	$7,000	$7,000	$7,000	$47,544
Avg. Age of Plant (years)	7.1	7.3	7.5	7.4	7.8	8.2	
Competitive Age of plant		7.1	7.1	7.1	7.1	7.1	
Competitive Capital ($000s)		$14,172	$14,172	$8,000	$11,000	$13,000	$61,744

The average age of plant is a key to determining the proper size of an organization's capital budget. Community Medical Center can establish an appropriate level of investment for competitive financial performance by plotting:

- Historical and projected average age of plant trends for its own facility.

- Comparative average age of plant trends for other competitive facilities.

Table 2-3 correlates the medical center's capital investment to its average age of plant, projected both at the currently budgeted level and at a level required to maintain Community Medical Center's competitive age of plant at 7.1 years. The medical center's five-year capital requirements will range from a minimum of about $47 million to about $61 million. If the organization can manage to remain competitive with a slowly increasing age of plant, as budgeted, the $47 million may be enough. The CEO of Community Medical Center feels that this minimum investment level and its corresponding average age of plant (8.2 years in 1997) will keep the organization in good standing, barring any unexpected changes in the competitive marketplace.

What Implications Do Capital Requirements Have on Operations?

Next we need to calculate the organization's total capital shortfall. You will remember:

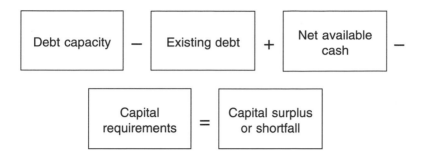

We already know that the organization's minimum capital requirements equal $47 million. The basic calculations presented in Tables 2-4 through 2-6 supply the other critical variables.

As shown in Table 2-4, Community Medical Center's net available debt capacity (debt capacity minus existing debt) is an estimated $23 million. This calculation assumes a minimum debt service coverage of 2.5 times. The medical center's maximum debt service is computed by dividing the cash available for debt service of $11.4 million by the minimum debt service coverage of 2.5 times. The maximum debt service of $4.58 million is then converted to total debt capacity by assuming an amortization period and an interest rate for new debt. In this case, the assumed amortization period was 30 years and the assumed interest rate was 7 percent. Table 2-4 illustrates an essential point, that gross debt capacity is affected by four independent variables: cash available for debt service, target debt service coverage, interest rate assumptions, and amortization period. It is essential to monitor debt capacity on a regular basis since all of these variables can change at any time, possibly causing a mate-

Table 2-4 Net Available Debt Capacity of Medical Center

1993 Cash Available for Debt Service	$11,461
Target Debt Service Coverage	2.5 times
Maximum Debt Service	$4,584
Total Debt Capacity	**$56,899**
(assuming 30-year amortization and 7.0% interest rate)	
Less Outstanding Long-Term Debt	$33,832
Net Available Debt Capacity	**$23,057**

rial increase or decrease in the organization's net debt capacity.

Another critical financial planning variable is the calculation of minimum cash reserves. This is a major issue for many healthcare organizations. How much cash is enough cash? How much cash will it take to compete in a rapidly changing delivery system and at the same time protect the creditworthiness of the organization? Table 2-5 demonstrates two methods of calculating the minimum level of cash reserves. Method one uses a "days cash on hand" target, while method two employs the "cushion ratio" to create an appropriate cash target.

The target "days cash on hand" of 100 and the target "cushion ratio" of four times were selected to reflect balance sheet relationships for an "average" "A" rated hospital. In this case, the suggested minimum cash reserves range from approximately $18.3 million to $20.6 million. In any case, Community Medical Center is currently far short of its cash reserve target.

Table 2-6 integrates all of the critical financial planning variables in a capital position analysis. This analysis compares the uses and sources of funds and calculates

Table 2.5 Calculation of Minimum Cash Reserve Requirements

Days Cash on Hand Approach	
1993 Cash Operating Expenses	$75,282,000
Expenses per day	$206,000
Target Days Cash on Hand	× 100 days
Minimum Cash Reserve	**$20,600,000**
Debt Capacity-Based Approach	
Debt Capacity	$56,889,000
Associated Debt Service	$4,584,000
Target Cushion Ratio	× 4 times
Minimum Cash Reserve	**$18,338,000**

1993 Actual Cash Reserve $2,584,000

the expected capital shortfall or, in unusual circumstances, a capital surplus. Subtracting the required uses of funds from the estimated sources of funds for Community Medical Center results in an estimated capital shortfall of approximately $60 million.

In other words, if the medical center intends to spend capital of $47.5 million and establish a minimum cash position of $18.3 million, it must first develop a plan to close the cash shortfall of $60 million during the next five years.

All of the analysis now leads to the critical financial planning question, What levels of organizational profitability over the next five years would be necessary to close the capital shortfall and permit the full implementation of Community Medical Center's competitive plan? The answer to this question is clearly the linchpin of the financial planning analysis and is summarized in Table 2-7.

Table 2-6   Capital Position Analysis

Uses	
Identified Capital, 1994-98	$47,544
Funding of Minimum Cash Position	18,338
(4 times annual debt service)	
Principal Payments on Existing Debt, 1994-98	14,877
Total	**$80,759**

Sources	
Existing Cash (1993 Cash and Marketable Securities	$2,584
and Board Designated Assets)	
Total Debt Capacity–1993	$56,889
Less: Approximate Nonproject Proceeds	33,832
Less: Approximate Nonproject Proceeds	4,611
Net Available Debt Capacity	18,445
Total	**$21,030**

Estimated Capital Shortfall ($59,729)

The model first converts the medical center's baseline projections into a capital allocation summary. The three cash margins listed in the summary distill all of the preceding analyses into specific levels of operating performance. Community Medical Center must achieve an average cash margin (bottom line + depreciation) of almost 12 percent over the five-year planning period to close the capital shortfall of $60 million. The medical center's projected cash margin of 14.2 percent will more than suffice, leaving the organi-

Table 2-7   Capital Allocation Summary of Cash Flow
**   Requirement**

1994–98 Cash Flow Requirements	$59,729
Projected Total Operating and Nonoperating Revenue	$500,256
Required Average Cash Margin to Meet Capital Needs	**11.9%**
1993 Actual Cash Margin	**9.8%**

zation some cash to spare for unexpected investment opportunities. But at the 1993 cash margin of 9.8 percent, Community Medical Center would have no hope of attaining the cash position it needs to meet both its balance sheet targets and the capital needs set forth in its strategic plan.

How Do Projected Baseline Results Compare with Minimum Required Profitability?

The next step is to test the reasonableness of the analytic outcome. If the capital shortfall can be closed by an average cash margin of 11.9 percent over the planning period, is it reasonable for the medical center to expect to operate at that level of profitability? Such a test can be provided first by the capable use of financial forecasts and then through the creative use of target and sensitivity analyses.

Table 2-8 summarizes the assumptions used to forecast the medical center's financial performance through the five-year planning period. The results of the baseline forecasts are summarized in Table 2-9.

When the baseline projection results in Table 2-9 were presented to the Community Medical Center Board, the reaction was twofold. First, the board recognized that improved financial operations at levels indicated by the "excess cash margin" would successfully close the capital shortfall. Second, the board recognized that the projections and their accompanying assumptions were optimistic and defined results that would require the medical center to greatly improve its financial performance. In other words, the board

Table 2-8   Baseline Forecast Assumptions

	1994 Inpatient	1994 Outpatient	1995 Inpatient	1995 Outpatient	1996 Inpatient	1996 Outpatient	1997 Inpatient	1997 Outpatient	1998 Inpatient	1998 Outpatient
Admissions	10,237		10,237		10,237		10,237		10,237	
Patient Days	66,252		65,589		64,934		64,284		64,641	
Outpatient Visits	94,553		102,117		108,244		114,739		120,476	
Inflation	8%		8%		6%		6%		5%	
Price Inflation	8%		7%		7%		6%		6%	
Reimbursement Inflation										
Medicare	2%	3%	2%	3%	2%	3%	2%	3%	2%	3%
Medicaid	5.5%	5.5%	4%	4%	4%	4%	4%	4%	4%	4%
Blue Cross	6.5%	95%	5%	90%	5%	90%	5%	90%	5%	90%
Commercial	Full Charges		Full Charges		Full Charges		Full Charges		Full Charges	
Other Operating Revenue	6%		6%		6%		6%		6%	

FTEs   Decrease from 1,303 in 1994 (5.27 average occupied beds) to 1,205 in 1998 (4.5 AOB)

Expense Inflation Rates:
Salaries   4% to 7% Inflation
Supplies   5% to 6% Inflation
Medical Fees   5% to 10% Inflation
Utilities   2% Inflation
Other   5% Deflation to 1% Inflation
Purchased Services   10% Deflation to Stable
Facilities   No Growth to 5% Inflation

	1994	1995	1996	1997	1998
Capital Expenditures	$13,672	$12,872	$7,000	$7,000	$7,000

Long-Term Debt $32.0 million by 1998; $13.0 million of additional debt is issued in 1994

Table 2-9   Baseline Projection Highlights

	1994	1995	1996	1997	1998
			($000s)		
Net Income (Loss)	$3,830	$4,510	$4,754	$6,344	$8,759
Unrestricted Cash Balance	$2,970	$3,987	$7,848	$14,241	$23,351
Operating Margin	3.7%	4.2%	4.0%	5.1%	6.6%
Excess Margin	4.3%	4.8%	4.8%	6.0%	7.8%
Debt Service Coverage	2.3×	2.5×	2.6ö	3.4×	4.2×
Capitalization Ratio	54%	49%	44%	40%	34%
Cushion Ratio	.5×	.7×	1.2×	2.6×	4.4×
Days Cash on Hand	14.1 days	18.1 days	33.7 days	59.2 days	93.2 days
Excess Cash Margin	12.0%	12.9%	13.6%	15.2%	17.2%

wanted to understand the overall risk involved, as
well as the risk to the financial plan of changing assumptions and scenarios, before committing to a specific financial strategy and operating plan.

What Are the Risk Points of the Financial Plan?

In this case, the medical center's board and senior management determined to test the sensitivity of the projected results to changes in five "what-if" scenarios:

1. What if admissions decrease 1 percent per year?

2. What if the medical center is forced to maintain
    its average age of plant at 7.1 years to remain
    competitive?

3. What if staffing levels increase from 4.5 full-time
    equivalents (FTEs) per adjusted occupied bed to
    5.0?

4. What if outpatient growth remains steady at 4
    percent instead of tapering from 8 to 5 percent?

5. What if the payer mix shifts, with a 1 percent
    increase in Medicare utilization and a corre-
    sponding 1 percent decrease in commercial
    payer utilization?

Comparing these operating scenarios to the baseline analysis, Table 2-10 quantifies the impact these
downside risks would have on Community Medical
Center's net income and cash projections. A decrease
in admissions will not alter the baseline significantly.
The need to raise competitive capital, on the other

Table 2-10 Downside Risk Analysis: Projected Impact of Selected Operating Scenarios ($000s)

Operating Assumption	Resultant 1998 Levels		Incremental Impact on 1998	
	Net Income	Unrestricted Cash	Net Income	Unrestricted Cash
Baseline	$8,759	$23,351	—	—
Admissions Decrease	$7,917	$21,765	($842)	($1,586)
Competitive Capital	$5,686	$7,665	($3,073)	($15,686)
Staffing Increases	$1,996	$3,413	($6,762)	($19,938)
Outpatient Growth of 4% per year	$6,873	$18,525	($1,885)	($4,826)
Payer Mix Shift	$8,410	$22,095	($348)	($1,256)

hand, will significantly reduce cash reserves. The medical center lacks the debt capacity to absorb a sudden increase in capital spending. Labor is the critical component of this risk analysis; in fact, the success of the organization may depend entirely on its ability to control labor costs. Outpatient growth, however, would have a minimal effect on projected levels of income and cash, as would a shift in payer mix. The risk analysis helps acclimate the board to changing market and operating conditions. Should any unexpected changes occur, decisionmakers will quickly understand the financial impact and can act swiftly to restore financial equilibrium.

Results

Community Medical Center's financial planning process leads its board and executives to four main conclusions:

1. Controlling operating expenses will be critical to the medical center's ability to deliver capital in support of its competitive strategies.

2. Strengthening the medical center's cash reserves should be the primary financial objective. A cash target of $18 million will help solidify the medical center's bond rating and hopefully maintain access to bond insurance.

3. Maintaining profitability while increasing incremental debt capacity is an essential strategy. A target excess cash margin of 11.9 percent over the next five years is critical to funding the medical center's full financial requirements.

4. Reviewing the debt and capital structure will be useful, since the current schedule of principal payments is reducing the medical center's cash and debt capacity positions.

The analyses that make up the financial plan have generated information that is rational, easy to understand, sophisticated, and immediately useful. The analyses will remain consistent and accurate throughout the five-year planning period. The findings permit the board and executive team to react quickly and correctly to changing circumstances.

Conclusion

The Community Medical Center case study highlights two chief benefits of the financial planning process. The financial plan provides the following:

1. A consistently reliable context for evaluating the organization's financial progress in strictly quantitative terms.

2. The flexibility, through computerized financial modeling techniques, to test the financial repercussions of pursuing new investments as strategic opportunities arise.

This combination of reliability and flexibility inspires confident decisionmaking and makes the organization highly adaptable to the changing health-care environment, lending the entire organization a strong sense of momentum. An organization with

sound financial planning practices is not easily diverted from its intended course.

CHAPTER 3

Mark L. Hall

Capital Deployment, Corporate Finance, and Constructive Decisionmaking

If an organization is successful in implementing the strategic financial planning process described in the previous chapter, it will possess the following:

1. A set of financial planning goals and objectives with specific targets relative to cash, capital expenditures, debt, and profitability levels.

2. An understanding of the financial dynamics of the existing operations sufficient to identify the key variables that it must manage to achieve the identified targets.

The above elements relate to the crucial task of *capital formation*, that is, putting the organization in a position where it has sufficient resources to support its strategic objectives.

What has been ignored up to now is the equally crucial task of wise *capital deployment*. The capital planning process can generate an extensive list of potential capital projects, but it is completely silent on whether any or all of the projects make sense for the organization. Clearly, the long-term success of the organization depends on its ability to make capital investment decisions that add to its future capital capacity and maintain or improve its creditworthiness.

In many organizations, the investment decision process focuses on specific projects in a serial fashion. A project concept grows out of a set of political and/or strategic considerations and develops a certain amount of momentum. The project is then handed off to the finance department, which "does the numbers." There is usually a fair amount of give-and-take (some of it productive, some not) as finance attempts to translate ideas into finite data. From those analyses come conclusions as to "feasibility," "affordability," and "return on investment," which become grist for additional deliberations.

This process worked reasonably well during the 1970's and '80s, but many organizations are beginning to notice that it is not up to today's challenges. Common complaints involve inconsistent methodologies and decision criteria and the lack of a level playing field among programs and projects. One response to these problems is to intensify the analytic effort brought to bear on specific projects. This is commendable but insufficient when the right attitudes and decisionmaking processes are not in place. The only way to improve the quality of investment decisions is to increase both the analytic efforts *and* the organizational rigor with which the decisions are made.

This rigor must be applied to two distinct sets of activities:

1. *Investment analysis,* which is concerned with determining the incremental effects that a specific initiative or project may have on the organization.

2. *Capital allocation,* which is the process by which the sum total of investment decisions is made.

The successful organization maintains a healthy degree of separation between the two processes.

The purpose of this chapter is to examine the analytic tools and organizational processes needed to support capital deployment decisions. After a discussion of the goals and theory of investment analysis, we present a case study that applies many of these principles. The chapter conclusion contains a discussion of the steps required for controlling the capital allocation process in an increasingly chaotic environment. The chapter is not a complete dissertation on the capital budgeting process, a subject about which entire textbooks have been written. Rather, it is intended as a guide to assist you in critically evaluating the relevant procedures in place at your organization.

Investment Analysis

Goals

Wise capital deployment starts with impeccable investment analysis. Successful organizations have developed a style and approach to investment analysis
that is consistent in attitude, methodology, and pace.
In this environment, any organization that deals with
strategic initiatives on an ad hoc basis is at a significant disadvantage.

The goals of investment analysis are fourfold:

1. *To define the project unambiguously.* Remember the
   old poem about the five blind men and the elephant? Depending on each man's point of
   "view," the elephant was described as being like
   a wall, a tree, a rope, a snake, or a spear. In our
   experience, this poem is often applicable to the
   project development process. It is amazing how
   far a project can proceed while different parts of
   the organization have fundamentally different
   visions of its scope and intent. Obviously, it is
   impossible to productively debate the merits of
   any initiative without substantive agreement on
   the facts.

2. *To identify the value that the project either adds to or
   subtracts from the organization.* There can be many
   reasons for pursuing a particular initiative, and
   financial return need not be the sole determi-
   nant. However, no project should be permitted
   to proceed if the organization is ignorant of its

impact on the organization's value and capital position.

3. *To delineate risk and success factors.* The elimination of cost-based reimbursement signaled the end of the usefulness of the feasibility analysis. In the new environment, decisions based on financial feasibility have been replaced by decisions based on educated risk taking. A financial forecast is interesting but is meaningless if it does not help the organization understand which variables need to be monitored and managed to ensure success.

4. *To provide a yardstick for review.* The concept of continuous quality improvement is applicable to the organization's decisionmaking process as well as to to its operations. The financially capable organization compares actual outcomes of accepted investments with budgeted results to assess progress and ensure the integrity of its analytic and decisionmaking processes.

Theory and Process

Successful investment analysis requires attention to four sets of activities:

1. Organization.

2. Business plan.

3. Net present value analysis.

4. Sensitivity analysis.

The fundamentals of each are described below:

Organization

A firm may have the latest hardware and software tools available, but organization, not analysis, is the initial step to first-class investment analysis and capital allocation. The key elements include:

1. *Identifying the expenditure threshold.* Many firms have established expenditure thresholds for capital projects, which trigger one or more levels of analysis or review. The approach taken says a lot about the firm. For example, one well-known for-profit firm was known to require executives of its local facilities to provide a detailed return-on-investment analysis for capital investments of $10,000 or more, whereas executives at a not-for-profit system with which we are familiar allocated discretionary budgets of a fixed amount to cover projects costing up to $300,000. Both represent extremes between which there is a happy medium. Beyond that, common sense dictates that there should be some reasonable relationship between the size and risk of the expenditure, the level of analysis effort required, and the level in the organization at which the review should take place. Be wary of situations in which there are so many projects under consideration that there is a push to raise the dollar threshold for analysis or to reduce the intensity of analysis.

2. *Appointing a project champion.* Once a major project is past the idea stage, it needs a champion who will take overall responsibility for definition, analysis, and implementation. In this environment, the traditional handoffs from planning, to finance, to construction, to operations provide many opportunities for misunderstandings and blurring of responsibilities. In many cases, the appropriate champion is the department head or executive who will have line responsibility for the project should it be implemented. When supported appropriately by planning and finance, this approach helps to ensure the development of a plan which is understood and considered reasonable by the executive who has to make it work.

3. *Defining the analytic framework.* A common mistake by senior management is the premature delegation of the analytic process. The successful organization will, at the outset, apply significant energy to revealing the key planning issues underlying the project and to identifying the level of analysis necessary to respond to them. This upfront attention always pays off in more focused and timely analysis. One way to focus the management team's thinking at this point is to explicitly consider specific alternatives to the initiative in question. In certain cases, the alternative is simply to not pursue the initiative. On the other hand, there may be other, potentially more attractive approaches that might otherwise be missed.

Business plan

The first task in any quest for either debt or equity to fund an entrepreneurial dream is the development of a business plan. A business plan should describe the idea and its financial consequences in sufficient detail to permit an investor to make an informed investment decision. Prudent use of organizational resources requires nothing less.

The successful organization displays the attitude, "If you can't write it down, you can't do it," and requires that business plans be developed and presented according to a consistent method and format. A complete business plan incorporates the following elements:

1. A project description that specifies facilities, equipment, services, location, and dollars.

2. A description of how the proposed initiative fits within the organization's current strategic development philosophy and mission.

3. A market assessment sufficient to give the reader a good sense of the dynamics of the market and its competitors as well as a rationale for volume, service, and revenue projections.

4. An implementation plan that delineates key tasks, dates, and challenges of implementation.

5. A five-year financial analysis. Given the proliferation of the personal computer and software technology, there is no excuse for a business plan not to have a full set of five-year financial

projections, including income statement, balance sheets, and statements of changes in financial position. There should be sufficient detail for the reader to understand the assumptions underlying the numbers, and the process should highlight the variables critical to the project's success. A first-class PC model should be used for appropriate "what-if" analysis. Depending upon the nature of the project at hand and its alternative, it may be appropriate to do a project-specific projection. On the other hand, if significant spillover or incidental effects have an impact on the core business, the best approach might be to develop the financial projections at the core business level using "project" and "nonproject" scenarios.

6. A well-defined exit strategy. Since it is impossible for everything to go right all of the time, it is essential that every major project have a strategy for modification and/or termination. It should identify appropriate warning signals and delineate the steps that would be taken to limit the organization's risk.

The business plan elements outlined above certainly seem unremarkable, but it is surprising how many important capital decisions are made without completing this basic documentation.

Net Present Value Analysis

The business plan provides the organization with an idea of the financial dynamics of the project at hand. Generally, these dynamics incorporate an upfront capital expenditure, followed by a start-up period during which time there may be financial losses, hopefully followed by a period of financial perform-ance which represents a return on the investment. The next question is whether the expected return is suffi-cient. Also unanswered is the question of how this project might compare financially to others under consideration, but different cash flow patterns inevita-bly make comparisons difficult. What is needed at this point is an analytic technique to distill the financial ebbs and flows of the project to a single value.

Net present value analysis is based on two princi-ples:

1. A dollar today is worth more than a dollar next year.

2. Higher risks require higher rewards.

Understanding present value requires a basic un-derstanding of the mechanics of compound interest. Start with a dollar. If that dollar is invested today at an interest rate of r, its value a year from now may be expressed as $\$1 \times (1 + r)$. If $r = 7\%$ (or .07), the future value of the dollar is $\$1 \times (1.07)$ or $\$1.07$. Left invested for another year, the dollar would be worth $\$1.07(1.07)$, or $\$1 \times (1.07)^2$. The generalized form for the future value of a present sum of money is thus $FV = PV(1 + r)^t$,

where

$$
\begin{array}{rcl}
FV & = & \text{Future value} \\
PV & = & \text{Present value} \\
r & = & \text{Interest rate} \\
t & = & \text{Number of time periods}
\end{array}
$$

By rearranging the above terms, it is possible to express the present value of a future cash flow as follows:

$$PV = \frac{FV}{(1+r)^t}$$

The present value of an investment decision that results in a series of future cash flows may be expressed as follows:

$$NPV = C_0 + \frac{C_1}{(1+r)} + \frac{C_2}{(1+r)^2} + \frac{C_n}{(1+r)^n}$$

where

NPV = Net present value

C_0 = Upfront expenditure associated with the investment

$C_1, C_2 \ldots C_n$ = Particular cash flows expected in particular periods

r = Interest (or discount) rate

As an example, assume that an investment of $50 now would yield cash flows of $25 per year for three years and that the discount rate is 10 percent. The NPV of that investment would be:

$$(\$50) + \frac{\$25}{1.1} + \frac{\$25}{(1.1)^2} + \frac{\$25}{(1.1)^3} = (\$50) + \$23 + \$21 + \$19 = \$13$$

In corporate finance theory, the decision rule is that the investment is acceptable if it has a positive NPV, since this means that the investment generates more than the opportunity cost of capital.

Because of its simplicity and reliability, the NPV approach is the most universally accepted means of valuation in corporate finance.

NPV analysis requires four elements:

1. An estimate of the upfront investment.

2. A forecast of free cash flows.

3. A cost of capital estimate.

4. A terminal value estimate.

Each of these is discussed below.

Upfront Costs

If the business plan has been properly constructed, the determination of the upfront costs (or C_0 in our formula) associated with the project in question should be reasonably uncomplicated. Costs such as building, equipment, and professional fees are obvious and should be covered in the project description. The trick here is to look beyond the obvious. The following rules are helpful:

- *Look only at incremental expenditures and ignore outlays that already have been made.* For example, the $500,000 spent on architectural and engineering fees last year is not germane to the final decision whether to build the facility this year. These outlays are referred to as sunk costs.

- *Do not ignore opportunity costs.* If, for example, the facility in question is to be built on land that could be sold for $400,000, the value of the land should be considered in the decision.

- *Consider working capital requirements.* A new service will require a basic inventory of supplies; operating expenses will need to be paid from cash reserves before patient collections become sufficient to carry these expenses on an ongoing basis.

Free Cash Flow

The concept of free cash flow ($C_1, C_2 \ldots C_n$ in our formula above) relates to how much cash is generated in a particular year that could be available to distribute to an investor. The classic manner of describing this is:

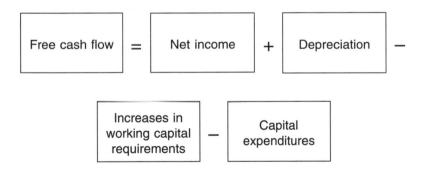

The financial forecasts prepared in the business plan should provide an excellent basis for developing this analysis over the projection period. These projections, however, should be examined critically to be sure they have been developed in a manner consistent with appropriate analysis.

The main considerations are to measure cash flow, not accounting profits, and to think incrementally. Neither depreciation nor allocation of existing corporate overhead should enter into the forecast. The key questions to answer are, What happens if we do the project? and What happens if we don't do the project? Remember that return on investment can be a function of reducing costs, maintaining market share, and/or creating new revenue sources. Other considerations include:

- *Ignore financing costs.* A fundamental tenet of corporate finance is the separation of the investment and the financing decision (known as the Separation Theorem). The cost of capital will be considered in a separate stage of this analysis, so the financial projections associated with the free cash flow analysis should assume that the project is financed with equity. There should, therefore, be no interest or principal payments in the free cash flow projections.

- *Explicitly estimate incidental effects.* For example, developing a surgicenter in an outlying part of the market area may cannibalize some existing outpatient surgery business, but it may also increase inpatient market share. If these effects are significant, they should be included in the analysis. This is an opportunity to quantify the strategic effects that are often the "x factor" in pushing a project ahead despite mediocre financial projections.

- *Incorporate inflation effects.* As will be discussed in greater detail below, the cost of capital is partly a function of market interest rates. In turn, interest rates reflect market expectations or inflation. To be consistent, the forecasts should reflect inflation expectations in revenues and expenses.

- *Remember ongoing capital requirements.* Do not forget the additional fixed and working capital requirements necessary to keep the investment operational.

Cost of Capital

Having developed forecasts of free cash flows, the next step is to determine by what rate the cash flows should be discounted. As stated earlier, if the investment is risky, it should have a higher expected return than funds invested in a relatively risk-free investment such as Treasury bills. The question is, How should the discount rate be set to account for the risk of a particular investment?

Much of the body of corporate finance theory centers on the issues of identifying the appropriate cost of capital (or discount rate) to be used in evaluating projects. Yet despite scholars' work and a considerable body of empirical evidence, there is still disagreement on which cost of capital should be applied to a given project. Similarly, within the healthcare community, there is a wide diversity of opinions as to how to calculate a not-for-profit organization's cost of capital.

A number of methods can be employed, but the conclusion common to all of the methods is that the real cost of capital is significantly higher than the cost of tax-exempt debt. This comes as a surprise to many executives, but this is amply demonstrated by the following examples.

General capital markets. This estimates the cost of capital for the capital markets as a whole. The formula is:

$$R_m = R_f + (R_m - R_f)$$

where

R_m	=	Market cost of capital
R_f	=	Risk-free rate, generally measured by the return on 30-year Treasury obligations
$R_m - R_f$	=	Historical spread between the market rate of return and the risk-free rate

Assuming that 30-year Treasury bonds (R_f) are trading at 6.5 percent and that the historical spread ($R_m - R_f$) is 8.3 percent, this equation results in an estimated cost of capital of 14.8 percent.

Firm-specific capital costs. Corporate finance scholars have also attempted to estimate the cost of capital to the healthcare industry by analyzing the behavior of stock prices for publicly traded healthcare firms.

The corporate model is often expressed as a variation of the general capital markets model.

$$R_c = R_f + \beta_c (R_m - R_f)$$

where

R_c	=	Corporate cost of capital
R_f	=	Risk-free rate (as described above)
$R_m - R_f$	=	Market risk premium (as described above)

β_c A factor (referred to as the firm's "Beta") that measures the risk of the firm in questions relative to the capital markets in general

The βs for individual stocks are published in the financial press on an ongoing basis. A β of 1 indicates that the stock in question is as "risky" as the stock market in general. Holding R_f and R_m - R_f constant from the previous example, and assuming a β for healthcare firms at 1.3, the above equation generates a cost of capital estimate of 17.2 percent.

Industry practice. Generally, investment bankers, corporate acquisition analysts, and financial consultants use a cost of capital factor of 15 to 20 percent for healthcare businesses, depending on the particular situation.

Debt market requirements. Given the historical dependence of the nonprofit hospital industry on public debt markets, the requirements of those markets are relevant. As discussed elsewhere, the rating agencies expect "A" rated organizations have sufficient cash flow to cover annual principal and interest on a loan by a factor of 2 to 2.5 times. Assuming that the project is 100 percent debt-financed over 30 years and that interest rates are in the 6 percent range, annual principal and interest would amount to about 7.25 percent of the total debt. The cash generated for debt service on an annual basis would, therefore, need to be 14.5 to 18.2 percent of the project cost.

Risk Analysis. One of the more interesting approaches in use in certain organizations is a risk classification approach to develop discount rates for specific projects. Each project is classified as high, medium, or low risk according to the following criteria:

1. The project requires that the organization generates market share from a new demographic or geographic market.

2. The project represents a new product or service for the organization.

3. The project requires management expertise, which the organization does not have and must recruit.

4. The project requires recruiting of more than five highly skilled or specialized personnel.

5. A strong competitor is present in the target marketplace.

Projects with one or fewer factors are classified as low-risk projects and are assigned a discount rate equal to twice the organization's long-term borrowing rate. Projects with two factors have a medium risk with a discount rate equal to two and one half times the borrowing rate. Projects with three or more factors have a discount rate of three times the borrowing rate.

Obviously, the determination of the appropriate discount rate is as much an art as a science. The major goal is to develop an approach that is defensible intellectually and to apply it consistently.

Terminal Value

A properly developed NPV analysis should incorporate some estimate of the investment's value after the original forecast period. This is referred to as its "terminal value." Depending on the project at hand, terminal value can account for 30 to 60 percent of the investment's total value. It therefore cannot be ignored. There are four basic ways to approach this calculation.

1. *No value.* This is probably a good approach for an item such as a computer, which is useful for a few years and then likely to become obsolete. It is probably much too conservative for an investment involving the development of a new service.

2. *Liquidation value.* This covers the anticipated sale value of the assets or the business on the open market at the end of the projection period.

3. *Annuity/perpetuity.* A commonly used approach is to assume that the investment will continue to generate free cash flow equal to that of the last projection period during a period ranging from one year to forever. This approach has some analytic appeal in that it is quite simple. For estimates involving a finite period (annuity), all you need is a calculator that has an annuity function. For estimates involving an indefinite time period (perpetuity), it is even simpler; divide the appropriate discount rate into the annual free cash flow.

4. *Growth perpetuity.* A common variation on the perpetuity approach is to incorporate an assumption about the rate of growth of free cash

flow after the project period. After all, if inflation causes revenues and expenses to increase
by 8 percent annually, then free cash flow
should grow by that rate as well. Although this
concept is technically correct, it is important to
note that the results of this method are extremely sensitive to the size of the growth assumptions. Accordingly, this approach should
be reserved for situations in which there is a fair
degree of confidence in those assumptions and
in the ongoing relationship between revenues
and expenses.

Whichever terminal value approach is employed, it
should be remembered that the terminal value accrues
to the project at the *end* of the forecast period. The
terminal value must therefore be discounted at the
same discount rate back to the beginning of the forecast period to define its present value. For example, if
the terminal value assumption is that the project will
be liquidated at the end of year five for $5 million and
the discount rate is 20 percent, the present value of
the terminal value is $5 million$/(1.2)^5$ or $2 million.

Sensitivity Analysis

The financial projections and the NPV analyses described in the previous pages are built on a set of
assumptions and judgments relative to the financial
dynamics of the project, the appropriate discount rate,
and the appropriate terminal value approach. Such
assumptions are subject to variability. As a result, no
investment analysis is complete without a series of

sensitivity analyses that address the potential for variability. In the days before the personal computer, this kind of analysis was time consuming. Today, the cost of examining incremental scenarios is relatively small. This obviously opens the door for all sorts of problems, not the least of which is the temptation to generate many scenarios and thus hamper decisionmaking. Scenario analysis can be effective only if it is focussed on determining what degree of variability in key assumptions and judgments can be tolerated before basic conclusions about the project would have to change. The financially competent organization knows how to draw this quantitative box around a project and use this information to derive an appropriate level of comfort and understanding.

A Case Study in Investment Analysis

A large community hospital, Midcity Hospital, operates in a medium-sized city with two significant competitors. The hospital enjoys a favorable reputation among the local medical profession, the community, and the emerging managed care plans. One of Midcity's specialties is its psychiatry and alcohol treatment services, which operate out of cramped but acceptable surroundings in the main hospital building. Owing to the quality of the staff, the hospital's behavioral services enjoy a good reputation among patients and payers and the inpatient units have high occupancy rates. The program director has two concerns relative to the future of the services. One is the lack of outpatient facilities, which he feels will be necessary in the managed care environment. The second is that he perceives significant service opportunities in women's and adolescent services. As a result, the organization's capital inventory carries a $6.0 million line item for the development and construction of a new freestanding behavioral medicine facility.

Organization

Given the magnitude of the expenditure, there is no doubt anywhere in the organization that this investment requires careful scrutiny. The obvious choice for project champion is the program director for behavioral services.

The analytic framework poses a challenge. The program director has an excellent idea as to the nature and scope of the proposed new facility; however, the fact that the existing in-house programs are currently profitable, albeit at risk, complicates the analysis somewhat. After deliberation, the management team agrees that the program director needs to develop two different business plans for the behavioral services. One would assume the development of the new facility, and the other would assume operation without making such a significant future investment.

Business Plan

The program director begins work on the business plans with representatives of the planning and finance department.

The business plan for the noninvestment alternative represents an end-game approach to the services. It involves the recognition that the current facilities and program complement, which are primarily inpatient oriented, are at a fundamental disadvantage in a marketplace that increasingly demands managed care. On the other hand, it is possible to take advantage of market position and pricing flexibility to minimize attrition in revenue. This, combined with strong expense control on a program-by-program basis, is expected to allow the organization to maintain a contribution margin at close to historical levels for the next five years, as delineated in Table 3-1.

The investment scenario requires a significant amount of effort to develop in detail. The new facility would increase treatment capacities. Plus, the program director has identified strong support for expanding Midcity Hospital's existing behavioral services among the local business and health plan communities. This, combined with the expected opportunities in adolescent and women's services, makes the team confident that this line of business has the potential to nearly double between 1993 and 1997.

The key question is whether this revenue growth would cover not just the incremental program-related expenses but also the overhead associated with opening and operating the new facility. Assessing this question requires the development of a fairly detailed operating plan that addresses the effects of the project on a number of hospital departments.

Summary revenue and contribution margin data for the investment scenario appear in Table 3-2.

Because the investment in the program would require a readjustment of aggregate revenue and ex-

Table 3-1   Contribution Outcomes of Noninvestment Scenario

	1993	1994	1995	1996	1997
Gross Revenue					
Psychiatry–Inpatient	$2,474	$2,138	$1,731	$1,870	$2,020
Psychiatry–Outpatient	569	392	422	453	487
Alcohol–Inpatient	2,951	2,680	2,352	2,541	2,731
Alcohol–Outpatient	1,122	1,085	987	1,061	1,140
Total	**$7,117**	**$6,296**	**$5,494**	**$5,976**	**$6,380**
Contribution Margin					
Psychiatry–Inpatient	$482	$389	$192	$262	$281
Psychiatry–Outpatient	49	(62)	(63)	(43)	(40)
Alcohol–Inpatient	1,818	1,682	1,500	1,651	1,784
Alcohol–Outpatient	189	144	177	141	163
Total	**$2,538**	**$2,154**	**$1,746**	**$2,011**	**$2,187**

Table 3-2 Contribution Outcomes of Investment Scenario

	1993	1994	1995	1996	1997
Gross Revenue					
Psychiatry–Inpatient	$3,864	$4,393	$5,140	$5,722	$6,180
Psychiatry–Outpatient	572	788	1,022	1,287	1,390
Alcohol–Inpatient	2,951	3,334	3,600	4,003	4,323
Alcohol–Outpatient	1,122	1,506	2,022	2,184	2,359
Adolescents	1,239	2,365	2,809	3,310	3,575
Women	578	1,100	1,452	2,081	2,247
Total	$10,327	$13,487	$16,046	$18,588	$20,075
Contribution Margin					
Psychiatry–Inpatient	$1,609	$1,797	$2,156	$2,208	$2,356
Psychiatry–Outpatient	37	156	211	314	344
Alcohol–Inpatient	1,775	2,015	2,147	2,289	2,491
Alcohol–Outpatient	182	438	445	414	491
Adolescents	590	1,369	1,609	1,698	1,839
Women	147	547	643	1,002	1,093
Facility Overhead	(1,787)	(1,817)	(1,969)	(2,004)	(2,104)
Total	$2,555	$4,507	$5,244	$5,923	$6,511

penses at the hospital, the alternative scenarios are evaluated through the preparation of a financial model for the entire hospital. Results of these financial projections are displayed in Table 3-3.

Table 3-3 indicates that the investment scenario represents fundamental changes in the business of the behavioral services:

1. Although 1997 gross program revenues improve by almost $14 million in the investment scenario, net revenues improve by only $10 million. This relates to the increased contractual allowances associated with the higher volume and managed care utilization.

2. With the exception of 1993, net income is consistently and significantly higher in the investment scenario.

3. Cash balances are lower in 1993 for the investment scenario, which reflects the initial $6 million investment and working capital requirements, but by 1996 this position reverses.

Table 3-3   Financial Projection Highlights ($ millions)

	1993	1994	1995	1996	1997
Revenue					
Investment	$147.1	$158.9	$169.9	$180.9	$192.5
Noninvestment	$144.3	$152.8	$161.1	$171.1	$182.0
Net Income					
Investment	$11.4	$13.8	$16.5	$18.1	$20.1
Noninvestment	$11.6	$11.9	$13.3	$14.3	$15.6
Cash Balance					
Investment	$38.8	$43.7	$52.0	$63.0	$76.8
Noninvestment	$44.9	$48.4	$54.0	$61.3	$70.6

Net Present Value

The financial projections provide an excellent point of departure for NPV analysis. The development of full financial statement projections simplifies the free cash flow calculations significantly, since initial capital, working capital, operating results, and ongoing capital are embedded in these projections.

Table 3-4 shows the derivation of the *incremental* free cash flow of the investment scenario compared with the noninvestment scenario.

Given the high-risk associated with new program establishment, the assumed growth and the vagaries associated with insurance coverage for these services, the finance department recommends and the management team accepts a high-risk discount rate of 20 percent for this project. This results in a present value calculation before consideration of terminal value (Table 3-5).

The data in Table 3-5 indicate a slightly positive NPV assuming no terminal value, which represents a strong result.

The next step is to determine which approach should be taken to estimate the terminal value of the investment scenario. One suggestion is to use perpetuity analysis. Other, more conservative members of the management team are concerned that events in the insurance industry may well eventually spell the end of all behavioral services. They suggest a liquidation approach assuming that the hospital might get 50 cents on the dollar for its original investment of $6 million. As shown in Table 3-6, these alternate approaches yield vastly different present value effects,

Table 3-4   Calculation of Free Cash Flow

Item	Begin	1993	1994	1995	1996	1997
				Year ($ millions)		
Ending Cash Balance, Investment	$34.0	$38.8	$43.7	$52.0	$63.0	$76.8
Ending Cash Balance, Noninvestment	40.0	44.9	48.4	54.0	61.3	70.6
Difference	(6.0)	(6.1)	(4.7)	(2.0)	1.7	6.2
Year-to-Year Change in Difference*	(6.0)	(0.1)	1.4	2.7	3.7	4.5

* Reflects incremental free cash flow

Table 3-5   Present Value Calculation

Year	Free Cash ($ millions)	Divided by Discount Factor	Equals Present Value ($ millions)
Begin	$(6.00)	1.0	$(6.00)
1993	(0.10)	(1.2)	(0.08)
1994	1.40	$(1.2)^2$	0.97
1995	2.70	$(1.2)^3$	1.56
1996	3.70	$(1.2)^4$	1.78
1997	4.50	$(1.2)^5$	1.81
Total			$0.04

which emphasize the sensitivity of the result to the terminal value approach taken.

Table 3-6   Terminal Value Alternatives

	Terminal Value ($ millions)	
	Future Value	Present Value
Perpetuity	$22.50	$9.04
Liquidation	$3.00	$1.21

The management team chooses the liquidation approach. Putting the two analyses together results in the following present value calculation:

Present value of free cash flow	$0.04 million
Present value of terminal value	$1.21 million
Present value	$1.25 million

For comparison purposes, if a discount rate of 15 percent were employed, the present value would be $2.6 million.

Subsequent discussions then focus on a less positive potential for the project. After consideration of key variables and related sensitivity analysis, the management team concludes that the incremental positive cash flows, with plausible assumptions, might be only 80 percent of what was projected in years 1994 to 1997. Terminal value would remain the same in this scenario.

The effect this has on the present value calculation is shown in Table 3-7.

Even with these assumptions, the project yields a small positive NPV. Based on the analyses, the management team decides to recommend approval of the building project to the hospital's board.

Table 3-7   Net Present Value Sensitivity Analysis

	$ millions	
Year	Free Cash	Present Value
Begin	(6.00)	(6.00)
1993	(0.10)	(0.10)
1994	1.12	0.78
1995	2.16	1.25
1996	2.96	1.42
1997	3.60	1.45
Terminal Value	3.00	1.21
Total		0.01

Capital Allocation

Crucial Elements

The management team in the preceding case conducted a well-executed and well-documented marginal project analysis. The decision that was made showed significant organizational maturity and judgment. On the other hand, this team, like many others, did not take the opportunity to put the decision in its most appropriate context. Excellent investment analysis needs to be accompanied by a capital allocation process that has the following elements:

1. An assessment of the short- and long-term capital constraints that the organization faces. At any time, the amount of resources that can be brought to bear is fixed. Knowledge of this constraint is essential.

2. A capital cycle that ensures that all worthy projects have a reasonably equal shot at consideration for funding. This concept is not based on democratic notions. Rather, it is based on the fact that a dollar spent on one initiative is no longer available to other projects. The organization that funds the first positive NPV project with complete analysis may find itself short of funds when a better opportunity arises.

3. A rationalization process for considering the aggregate effects of project decisions on the financial position and risk profile of the organization.

A word of caution—although many of the above steps can be supported through quantitative analysis, capital allocation remains an inherently messy process. To be successful, it must recognize the following:

1. Capital allocation is a competitive process, but it is best accomplished through a collaborative management and organizational style.

2. Governing and disciplining the process is hard; excessive compromise tends to defeat the purpose of the exercise and undermine confidence in the credibility of the allocation process.

3. The statistical methods, data base, and software tools used must be beyond challenge. If the quantitative analysis is discredited, the entire allocation process disintegrates. This requires investment in good tools and in developing an organizationwide understanding and comfort with such tools.

Defining the Capital Constraint

As indicated above, at any one time, each organization faces a limit on its capital resources; this limit is determined solely by its current operations, debt structure, and cash position. Improvements in operations resulting from today's investment decisions may produce more discretionary capital in the future but cannot affect the present. The myth that good projects generate their own capital is widespread. Likewise, the quest for "creative financing" often diverts time and attention from the real issues. The organization that does not understand its limits cannot make informed or timely decisions. On the other hand, a keen understanding of limits often helps an organization focus and economize on the effort used in the project development process. Once the capital constraint has been identified, the list of potential (and often dubious) projects shrinks accordingly. If the constraint is not clear, the organization may waste energy on ideas that have no chance at implementation.

The beginning point is to ask the simple question, What level of dollars are we reasonably sure we can provide to support the organization's development over a defined period? The evaluation issues relate to the organization's credit position and the risks that it is willing to take.

1. How much can we and should we borrow?

2. What level of cash can be generated from operations in uncertain times?

This process can work fairly simply if the organization has taken the effort to create sufficient confidence, understanding, and consensus in the financial planning process. The first two steps are as follows:

1. Confirm the targets for cash, debt service coverage, and debt-to-capitalization ratios established in the financial plan and translate them into annual goals.

2. Reconfirm the organization's debt capacity based on current-year operations and identify a five-year financial projection scenario to which the organization can commit.

Having accomplished the above, it is possible to construct a table similar to Table 3-8.

The analysis in Table 3-8 provides a reliable means of estimating capital availability. It is based on policy decisions to limit external borrowing to a predetermined level and an annual commitment to build cash

Table 3-8   Determination of Five-Year Capital Spending Pool

	Year 1	Year 2	Year 3	Year 4	Year 5	Total
Sources of Cash						
Revenues over Expenses	$6,000	$7,000	$7,000	$9,000	$11,000	$40,000
Depreciation/Amortization	7,000	7,000	7,000	7,000	7,000	35,000
Debt Proceeds	0	20,000	0	0	0	20,000
Fund Raising	2,000	2,000	2,000	2,000	2,000	10,000
Total	15,000	36,000	16,000	18,000	20,000	105,000
Uses of Cash						
Principal Payments	1,500	1,500	1,500	1,500	1,500	7,500
Additions to Working Capital	1,400	1,500	1,600	1,700	1,800	8,000
Contribution to Cash Reserves	3,300	2,500	2,200	2,500	2,500	13,000
Previously Committed Capital	5,000	0	0	0	0	5,000
Available Capital	**3,800**	**30,500**	**10,700**	**12,300**	**14,200**	**71,500**
Total	15,000	36,000	16,000	18,000	20,000	105,000

reserves to maintain a certain credit profile. It is not arbitrary or capricious. It may take a little while for certain parts of the organization to understand the allocation process, but it is necessary to persevere. There may be questions such as, Can't we squeeze another $5 million out of this somehow? and What about moving some of the financial capacity of 1998 into 1996? These questions represent fine-tuning issues that should not be addressed until there is agreement on the baseline parameter. Once these questions stop, the focus of the allocation process will become sharper.

Capital Cycle

Having determined the extent of available capital, the next question is how to allocate capital among competing uses. The previous sections of this chapter have dealt extensively with documentation and analysis requirements, but such analysis is ultimately useless without adequate attention to logistics, governance, and process issues. There are many ways to organize these activities, but effective capital allocation processes center around two principles:

1. There needs to be a capital cycle, to which the organization explicitly adheres. It is impossible to make good decisions among projects unless each project is presented in a comparable manner and at the same time. Some organizations time the capital cycle to coincide with the budget cycle; some find that keeping the process on different cycles allows more energy and at-

tention for decisionmaking. Some organizations use an annual cycle; others batch their decisions every six months. The point is to develop a cycle that works and to stick with it. Capital decisions deserve the same level of formality and structure as those surrounding the operating budget.

2. The mechanism for governing the process needs to be crystal clear. Almost anything can work so long as it is explicit and consistent. One religious healthcare system uses an annual CEO forum to consider and rank major strategic initiatives. At a freestanding hospital, a group of key physicians and senior executives perform this function and present a recommendation to the CEO and, ultimately, to the board. This kind of process might be threatening to a CEO who is used to allocating resources depending on the political vagaries of the moment. On the other hand, a murky decision process produces alienation and disaffection in the management ranks as well as the inevitable misappropriation of valuable capital to projects that are not analytically or financially worthy.

Project categorization and global allocation

Capital expenditures generally fall into one of the following categories:

1. Routine expenditures for repair and/or replacement.

2. Major expenditures relating to legal, safety, or regulatory requirements. Projects in this category include boiler and/or roof replacement, asbestos removal, and the like.

3. Major expenditures relating to significant strategic initiatives, such as starting a new service, building a medical office building, or replacing a cardiac catheterization lab.

4. Expenditures that, by their size and/or scope, have the potential to fundamentally alter the nature of the organization. Such expenditures might be the acquisition of an HMO or the development of a replacement facility.

These categories can be used to support an annual global allocation process, which identifies a threshold and establishes a budget for nonreviewable projects; sets a budget for mission-driven capital; and delineates spending requirements for legal, safety, and regulatory related projects. With these budgets established, the remainder is what is left over for strategic capital expenditures.

In any discussion of the mechanics of the global allocation process, the question that inevitably arises is, What happens if there's no money left over for strategic capital? In this case, one hopes that putting the global process through another iteration reduces the allowance for "entitlement" projects. If that doesn't help, the organization is left with an early warning signal, which the intelligent management team heeds immediately. One instructive exercise is to review past capital decisions to determine the histori-

cal amounts of capital actually spent on strategic initiatives. If expenditures for strategic initiatives routinely amount to a small portion of total expenditures,
the future of the organization is clearly in question.

Project ranking

Effective processes for project ranking consider standard corporate finance theory as a point of departure.
This body of theory is based on the maxim that the
role of the corporation is to maximize shareholder
value. This means that (1) no negative present value
investments are selected and (2) all positive net present value investments are selected, unless there are
constraints on available capital (in which case, the
combination of investments that maximize value
within the capital constraint is selected).

Not-for-profit healthcare organizations cannot be
guided solely by these principles because their mission is to serve the community, not to generate profits.
Therefore, not-for-profit organizations need to aug-
ment these criteria to take into account service, community, and mission priorities.

Many Catholic healthcare systems have been particularly interested in developing alternative models
for capital allocation, especially as these processes relate to mission and the cross-subsidization of capital
between operating units. Some systems have established weighting structures, the complexity of which
varies significantly, to capture mission, strategy, and
financial issues in a composite ranking. These systems
approve projects down the list until they reach the
capital constraint for that cycle.

Regardless of the weighting process, all the truly effective ranking procedures have one thing in common: a single table that lists the projects in descending order of NPV. An example is shown in Table 3-9.

This table becomes an important touchstone no matter what process is used to arrive at composite rankings, since it helps to provide unambiguous insight into the following considerations:

1. When considered as a whole, does this list of preferred projects have a positive or a negative NPV? In other words, by selecting this list of projects, is the organization adding to or detracting from its value? Clearly, no organization can carry a series of investment decisions that adversely affect its value.

2. What positive NPV projects have been left on the planning table? It is essential to understand that accepting projects with positive values now will help ensure the organization's mission in the future.

Rationalization and Risk Analysis

At this point, it is useful to come back to three simple financial imperatives:

1. Create capital capacity more rapidly than you expend it.

2. Remain creditworthy.

3. Don't run out of cash.

Table 3-9   Project Inventory

Project	Cost		Financial Return	
	FY 1994 Project Cost ($000s)	Total Cost ($000s)	NPV ($000s)	Key Assumptions
Surgicenter/MOB	$7,000	$7,500	$18,963	Low risk
				Volume projections appear conservative but could be impacted by competitor freestanding surgicenter
Add Outpatient Catheterization Lab	$1,400	$1,400	$9,362	Low risk
				Incremental volumes assume partial recapture of lost/diverted referrals
Initiate Cardiac Surgery	$533	$708	$5,545	Moderate risk
Towers Club Renovation	$2,800	$2,800	$3,141	Moderate risk
				Slower fill-up and/or different sales mix would negatively impact financials

Continued on next page

Table 3-9   Project Inventory (continued)

| Project | Cost | | Financial Return | |
	FY 1994 Project Cost ($000s)	Total Cost ($000s)	NPV ($000s)	Key Assumptions
North Campus Ambulatory Care/MOB	$22,793	$33,660	$2,467	Moderate risk Financials assume incremental inpatient revenues related only to Cancer Treatment Center Certificate of Need required
Perinatal	$650	$650	$881	Low risk. Should assist in regaining 100+ scheduled inductions per year that have been lost to competitors
Special Procedures Room	$980	$980	$747	Low risk
Electrophysiology Lab	$1,000	$1,000	$718	Moderate risk Nationally recognized electrophysiology specialist has been recruited to initiate program

Continued on next page

Table 3-9   Project Inventory (continued)

| Project | Cost | | Financial Return | |
	FY 1994 Project Cost ($000s)	Total Cost ($000s)	NPV ($000s)	Key Assumptions
Assisted Living Facility (joint venture with developer)	$1,000	$5,300	$238	Moderate risk Venture structure must be negotiated; need to address control issues and financing Represents new model not currently available in market
Primary Care Physician Network	$1,366	$1,366	($490)	Moderate Risk Practice management expertise must be obtained MD acquisition targets may be aggressive
Physician/Hospital Integration	$2,000	$2,000	($1,173)	Moderate risk Effective management of practice costs is critical for positive cash flow (negative cash flow assumed through year 3 of projections)

It is possible to make a series of positive NPV decisions, have the business plans materialize, and still go
out of business. The first step in managing this risk is
to understand it.

This requires the integration of the results of the
financial planning and capital allocation processes
completed thus far in a manner that increases the organization's decisionmaking confidence. The steps are
as follows:

1. Start with the updated baseline financial projections used to calculate the capital constraint.

2. Incorporate the results of the selected investment set into these financial projections to create
   a single set of consolidated projections.

3. Based on the above steps and on the nature of
   the projects at hand, identify a preliminary borrowing strategy. Ideally, this should identify the
   amount and type of borrowing anticipated to
   support the investment strategy over the next
   couple of years. It may be appropriate to consult
   with the organization's financial adviser and/or
   investment banker in this matter.

4. Reflect the borrowing strategy in the updated
   financial projections; this will become the organization's new baseline financial projections.

The risk assessment relative to this new baseline
should focus on the following areas:

1. *Financial profile.* Does the revised baseline exhibit
   an adequate financial profile? Are cash reserves,

debt service coverage, and leverage ratios acceptable on a year-by-year basis? Do they exhibit stable or generally improving trends? A financial plan that shows declining trends without the possibility of improvement is a sure route to a rating downgrade.

2. *Core risk.* How sensitive are the results to variability of the assumptions of the core business? Does the organization have adequate financial altitude, or should final adjustments be made to base-year core expenses or to the capital expenditure plan?

3. *Project risk.* How sensitive is the whole to the results of the project? If a commitment entails significant risk, the organization must understand and prepare proactive strategies to manage that risk. For example, a multihospital system was in the process of developing a new facility. The business plan for the facility incorporated assumptions about the rate at which utilization would build at that site. The risk analysis determined that, if the utilization did not materialize according to schedule, the system could find itself with an unacceptably low cash position. The solution to this was to secure a line of credit before the problem materialized.

4. *Portfolio risk.* At what level does the investment set need to perform? If most projects need to succeed as projected to keep the organization in business, the planning tolerances may be too

tight. Better to plan for a less-than-perfect bat-
ting average.

5. *Capital formation.* What happens to the organization's incremental debt capacity on a year-to-
year basis? Will the organization be able to respond to as yet unidentified opportunities?

The final steps are to modify the plan based on the
preceding considerations and to finalize implementation decisions and timetables.

Monitoring of Strategic Initiatives

One of the attributes of effective organizations is the
degree to which the consequences of decisions are
made visible throughout the organization. The capital
allocation processes described above encourage a rigorous business planning process and the development
of an annual operating plan.

Do not miss the opportunity to close the planning
loop by installing a post-implementation monitoring
process for the strategic initiatives approved in each
cycle. As practiced by a number of organizations, this
process involves the comparison of actual versus
planned results through a five-year program of annual submittals. This report is often reviewed in context with the setting of the capital constraint and the
ranking of projects in the current cycle.

Conclusion

The analytic and decisionmaking processes described in this chapter reflect the following philosophical principles:

1. In an environment of scarce resources, competition among ideas on how to best allocate these resources is usually helpful so long as the rules for this competition are delineated and followed.

2. Financially driven decisionmaking is not inconsistent with mission-driven healthcare. It does, however, require that the dollars allocated to mission be explicitly identified and kept in a balance consistent with the long-term financial health of the organization.

3. The role of financial analysis is to facilitate decisionmaking; it is not an end in itself. This places a heavy burden on the nonfinancial side of the management team to identify questions that require financial analysis. It puts an equal and opposite burden on the finance department to determine the level of analysis necessary and to structure and present the analyses in a coherent fashion.

4. The fundamental responsibility of management is to manage. Even the best decisionmaking supported by the most competent financial analysis may be proved wrong by external circumstances. The ability to disengage from bad deci-

sions is at least as important as the ability to make good ones.

The quantitative techniques described in this chapter are not extraordinary in that they require skills and personal computer software and technology that are readily available. The critical success factors are the willingness and the ability to use these techniques constructively to help chart and modify your organization's course.

CHAPTER 4

Therese L. Wareham

Analysis of Acquisitions

Strong financial performers enjoy a marked strategic advantage over their less creditworthy rivals, especially in this era of mergers and acquisitions. A healthcare organization that has established a strong capital position is better fit to expand or reconfigure operations, stave off competitors, and invest in the future. But even the most creditworthy organization must back up its financial prowess with informed decision-making and excellent executive judgment. The leadership team must be fed a constant supply of fresh, accurate, and readily interpretable information to champion the organization's strategic causes in a sometimes hostile marketplace.

Of all the ventures a financially capable healthcare organization may pursue, none is more demanding than an acquisition. The financial plan provides a

solid foundation upon which to build such a successful acquisition strategy. Buying another facility will
test the mettle of an organization's strategic vision
and analytic skill. But with proper financial guidance
and sound modeling practices and techniques, the
process of identifying acquisition opportunities, negotiating a price, and closing the deal can be far less
trying. The financially capable healthcare organization can assess its acquisition opportunities in quantitative terms and then apply those rigorous analyses to
gain the upper hand in negotiations.

In this chapter we present case studies of three acquisition scenarios:

1. *Buy and Operate*—in which a large tertiary care
   medical center considers acquiring a neighboring women's hospital as a means of establishing
   obstetric services.

2. *Buy and Close*—in which a midsized acute care
   hospital examines the ramifications of buying
   out a smaller local competitor to regain lost market share.

3. *Buy and Reconfigure*—in which a system-owned
   rural regional provider decides whether to acquire the facility of its only direct competitor to
   house expanding ambulatory surgery and inpatient rehabilitation programs.

Each of these acquisition scenarios demonstrates
the critical importance of thoughtful strategic decisionmaking informed by rigorous financial analysis.

Guiding Principles

Beyond the basic principles of corporate finance, every acquisition analysis should abide by three guiding principles:

1. *Keep investment decisions separate from financing decisions.* The buying decision—a purely strategic consideration—should not be complicated by the choice of cash or debt financing vehicles. The decision to invest is made first without capitalization assumptions. The investment decision is tested afterward against financing realities.

2. *Analyze the value of the operations to you, not to the seller or a third party.* The objective of the acquisition is to determine the amount you would pay for an operation to realize a break-even return. From there, you can negotiate a mutually acceptable purchase price.

3. *Focus on cash flows.* The value of a potential acquisition should be calculated using the discounted cash flow method. The issues and approach are as reviewed in Chapter 3. Bricks and mortar used for a single purpose do not create value in and of themselves. Instead, continuing value is created through the business performed within the bricks and mortar. Expected future cash flows will ultimately determine the value or purchase price of a targeted acquisition. Traditionally, a multiple of historical cash flow provided an acceptable value. Given the volatility of financial performance in the healthcare indus-

try due to reimbursement changes and impending healthcare reform, future cash flow generation is the key. Most sellers sell because something has just recently gone wrong or is expected to deteriorate; utilization may have decreased, for instance. Therefore, the focus should be on creating an accurate forecast of five years of incremental free cash flow from the potential acquisition, defined as follows:

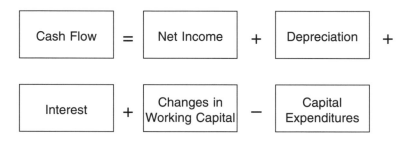

These future five years' free cash flows are then discounted back to today's dollars using a factor that represents the certainty or uncertainty of realizing those cash flows.

The discount rate, or cost of capital, selected should reflect the rate of return expected from funds invested at a particular level of risk. Although this is a rate that can be specifically calculated for many for-profit corporations, the selection of a discount rate for not-for-profit institutions involves a series of educated guesses. In summary, the discount rate applied:

- Is an adjustment to the current market risk-free rate of return.

- Will be higher for riskier ventures.

- Should reflect the cost of capital of the seller, not the buyer.

- Should not be less than the long-term debt borrowing rate of the seller.

Assuming that the business being purchased is expected to survive beyond five years, then the value of the operation should incorporate some estimate of those continuing cash flows. As discussed in Chapter 3, one common approach to calculating this terminal value is known as the perpetuity method. This is as simple as dividing the discounted cash flow from year five by the discount rate. You then discount this value to the present and add it to the sum of the discounted cash flows from the five-year forecast.

Note that hard assets should only be considered later, when the transaction structure is actually being defined. Property, plant, and equipment do not figure in this analysis phase of the acquisition.

The practical application of these guiding principles will figure prominently in each of our three case studies.

A Case Study: Buy and Operate

A 650-bed tertiary care Catholic hospital that offers virtually all services but obstetrics (OB) wants to build or buy a facility to house a new OB department. Building a brand-new facility, the leadership team has determined, would cost $20 million. Another appealing option is to purchase the facility across the street, a 200-bed women's hospital owned by a for-profit chain.

Senior management must decide whether buying the neighboring women's hospital is the best strategy and, if so, how much the hospital should pay to acquire it.

Issues to Consider

Before purchasing a business that you intend to continue operating, several important considerations come into play. In this acquisition scenario, the prospective buyer researches and addresses the following questions:

- *Medical staff.* Are the medical staff members of the women's hospital properly credentialed? What other options might physicians pursue in the local market if the facility is purchased? Will the doctors be loyal and remain on staff after the change in ownership? Who would replace the physicians who leave?

- *Demographics.* What are the demographic trends? Will there be an adequate population of women of childbearing age?

- *Contracts.* Are the prospective seller's managed care contracts good arrangements? What are the implications of any contracts that might be lost or gained in the transaction? Contracts that will transfer with the sale must be considered an integral part of the whole package.

- *Cannibalization/overlaps.* Will procedures now performed at one or the other hospital be performed exclusively at one or the other site after the sale? Since the buyer is a Catholic hospital, will it forfeit an OB business that does not fit its religious mission? Abortion and sterilization services comprise six diagnosis-related groups (DRGs) that the purchasing organization will not perform.

• *Staffing*. Will the buyer have to provide and staff services currently provided by the seller's parent chain? What kinds of staffing synergies between the neighboring facilities can be expected? The buyer should not pay for services or staff that it will not receive in the sale or will not need after the sale.

• *Economics*. What will be the economic arrangements between the facilities in terms of insurance and other types of operating expenses?

• *Working capital*. What are the seller's working capital needs? The buyer should be prepared to provide the acquired organization about 60 days of working capital.

Any of these issues can dominate the analysis and negotiation of a facility sale. In this case, managed care contracts become the buyer's chief concern and the central thrust of the negotiating process.

Approach

The hospital's acquisition analysis proceeds in five steps:

1. Define the cash flows that the hospital expects the acquired obstetrics operation to generate.

2. Determine the key variables of vulnerability, that is, the operating assumptions that pose certain risks.

3. Run the key variables through sensitivity analyses to quantify the changes in cash flows under various risk scenarios.

4. Using the discounted cash flow method, calculate the value of those risk-adjusted cash flows.

5. Define a range of values for the new OB operation based on the varying cash flows.

To define expected cash flows, the buyer gathers as much utilization and financial data as possible—at least one to two years of historical data, particularly utilization and revenue by payer. In this case, the facilities sign confidentiality agreements, so getting the necessary data is not a problem. Otherwise, public information, such as Medicare cost reports, is available at the state and local levels. In many states, certain utilization and financial information is published quarterly.

Year-to-date financial statements were very important since changing financial performance was significantly affecting the value of the business being acquired and, therefore, the negotiating posture.

The buyer selects three key variables of vulnerability—no utilization growth, low utilization growth, and high utilization growth—and assigns probabilities to each to calculate a range of values under the various scenarios and costs of capital, as shown in Table 4-1. After examining these scenarios and their corresponding range of values, and considering demographic data and other issues, the buyer's management team concludes that the women's hospital essentially is driven by inpatient utilization, which probably can be expected to remain flat. For the buyer, the most immediately convincing scenario is a 60 percent probability of no utilization growth. So, as shown in Table 4-1, the buyer decides on a purchase offer of about $41 million.

The seller insists on valuing its facility at six times the previous year's cash flow, or $45 million. But this price does not take into account:

- Procedures that are nonallowable and would be lost to a Catholic buyer.

- The seller's poorer financial performance in the current year.

- Recent utilization decreases.

- The proprietary chain's plan to substantially reduce reimbursement under its contract with its own managed care plan, which covers 18 percent of the seller's patient days and is due for renewal and renegotiation.

The buyer surely faces other risks in this transaction, but the allure of an ideally suited facility just across the street justifies further negotiation. The buyer returns to its financial model and prepares a counterproposal for the seller.

Table 4-1   Buy and Operate: Sensitivity of Values Based on Three Utilization Assumptions

	Probabilities	Values ($000s)		
		12.7% Cost of Capital	14.5% Cost of Capital	Average
No Growth Scenario:	100%	$31,867	$28,387	$30,127
Low Growth Scenario:	100%	$58,944	$51,284	$55,114
High Growth Scenario:	100%	$65,241	$56,605	$60,923
No Growth Scenario:	33.3%			
Low Growth Scenario:	33.3% ⟩	$52,017	$45,425	$48,721
High Growth Scenario:	33.4%			
No Growth Scenario:	60%			
Low Growth Scenario:	20% ⟩	$43,957	$38,610	$41,284
High Growth Scenario:	20%			
No Growth Scenario:	20%			
Low Growth Scenario:	60% ⟩	$54,788	$47,769	$51,279
High Growth Scenario:	20%			
No Growth Scenario:	20%			
Low Growth Scenario:	20% ⟩	$57,307	$49,897	$53,602
High Growth Scenario:	60%			

Note: "Average" cost of capital is approximately 13.6%

Negotiations

Approaching the bargaining table, the buyer comes armed with new analyses and a solid negotiating posture. The analyses, shown in Tables 4-2 through 4-4, put stock in the buyer's argument that $45 million is a reasonable price for the women's hospital, but only if the seller's managed care contract and total volumes are part of the deal. Table 4-2 shows the argument in a nutshell: without the seller's contracted managed care volumes, the value of the women's hospital is only about $30 million, $11 million less than the buyer's baseline figure of $41 million. Table 4-3 details the value of this $11 million contract in terms of patient volumes and revenues.

The buyer argues that it is willing to pay an 8.9 percent premium, or $4 million (the seller's $45 million asking price minus the buyer's $41 million valuation) for the new facility, but not 33.3 percent, or $15 million ($45 million minus the no-contract baseline of $30 million). Without the $11 million contract, the hospital will pay the same 8.9 percent premium over the $30 million baseline, or about $32.7 million.

To convince the seller that its logic is sound and its analysis is fair, the buyer projects both organizations' future performance assuming that the proposed ac-

Table 4-2 Buy and Operate: Summary of Valuation Analyses

Contemplated Purchase Price	$45,000,000
Baseline Financial Valuation	$41,000,000
Appraised Value of Plant, Property, and Equipment	$35,000,000
Financial Valuation Excluding Seller's Managed Care Volumes	$30,000,000

Table 4-3   Buy and Operate: The $11 Million Managed Care Contract

FY 1992 Volumes:	1,277 Inpatient Discharges
	5,360 Patient Days
	3,098 Outpatient Visits
FY 1992 Revenues:	$10,422,000 Gross Revenues
	$ 3,589,000 Net Revenue

quisition is unsuccessful. Its analysis assumes that the women's hospital would operate at the optimistic patient volumes suggested by the seller, increasing its value to $49 million. But the Catholic hospital would open its own obstetrics unit and, in the first year, take an estimated 1,200 admissions away from the women's hospital. The loss of admissions each year would reduce the value of the women's hospital to $26.3 million. These projections rather convincingly portray the facility and contract package deal as the seller's best possible strategic move.

Because the buyer has done its homework so thoroughly, negotiators are able to produce the analysis with which they can fix the price and close the sale. Table 4-4 shows how the purchase price is affected by the two critical terms of the $11 million contract: discount reimbursement from charges and contract exclusivity. With this analysis, the buyer communicated the fairness of the counteroffer to the seller and suggested support for a higher price assuming improved contract terms.

Table 4-4 Buy and Operate: Analysis of Seller Contract on Valuation ($000s)

Discount from Charges	2 Years Exclusivity		3 Years Exclusivity		5 Years Exclusivity
67%	Lose 12% Yr 1 Lose addl 3% Yr 2 Lose addl 2% Yr 3	$39,384	Lose 12% Yr 1 Lose addl 3% Yr 2	$39,627	$41,000
65%	Lose 12% Yr 1 Lose addl 3% Yr 2 Lose addl 2% Yr 3	$40,800	Lose 12% Yr 1 Lose addl 3% Yr 2	$41,085	$41,847
60%	Lose 20% Yr 1 Lose addl. 7% Yr 2 Lose addl. 5% Yr 3	$43,640	Lose 20% Yr 1 Lose addl 7% Yr 2	$44,482	$46,515
55%	Lose 25% Yr 1 Lose addl 11% Yr 2 Lose addl 5% Yr 3	$46,191	Lose 25% Yr 1 Lose addl 11% Yr 2	$47,603	$51,184
50%	Lose 30% Yr 1 Lose addl 15% Yr 2 Lose addl 5% Yr 3	$48,174	Lose 30% Yr 1 Lose addl 15% Yr 2	$50,275	$55,852
45%	Lose 35% Yr 1 Lose addl 20% Yr 2 Lose addl 10% Yr 3	$48,901	Lose 35% Yr 1 Lose addl 20% Yr 2	$52,396	$60,520

Results

Through shrewd negotiations informed by rigorous analyses, the buyer achieves the following excellent results:

- The seller agrees to renew its managed care contract for five years at existing terms.

- The buyer acquires the women's hospital for $45 million.

- Staffing levels following the acquisition are even better than anticipated.

- Utilization initially falls off more sharply than expected (because the ban on nonallowable procedures led some physicians to practice elsewhere) but is slowly returning.

In short, the hospital has used thorough financial planning and analysis to successfully negotiate not only the price but the terms and financial implications of an acquisition, which is now an integral component of its healthcare services.

A Case Study: Buy and Close

A 430-bed acute care hospital with excess inpatient capacity has been steadily losing market share to several competitors and is seeking to rebuild its patient base. Although the hospital is located on a constricted campus, strategic planners have identified the need to expand psychiatric services and start up a rehabilitation or skilled nursing facility. A 170-bed hospital 10 blocks away looks ideal for this purpose.

The financial planners must decide whether the hospital can recapture its lost market share through the acquisition of the nearby facility and whether the acquired facility would be an appropriate space in which to provide the alternative services efficiently and cost-effectively.

Issues to Consider

Buying and closing an institution has stronger implications than does a buy-and-operate scenario. Patients and staff will be displaced, not merely placed under new management and ownership.

In this case, the buyer considers several key issues:

- *Medical staff.* How much patient volume will the seller's medical staff actually shift to the buyer? What about specialty mix? In this service area, physicians practice at several medical centers. If the seller's physicians are not attracted to the buyer's facility, they could just as easily move their admissions to other local competitors.

- *Demographics.* What are the trends in the market? Are there patients whom the buyer especially wants to attract?

- *Staffing.* What effects might the incremental volume have on the buyer's staffing complement?

- *Closure expenses.* How much will it cost to pay laid-off employees their severance, provide insur-

ance and security for an empty building, and
cover other closure expenses?

- *Outpatient activity.* Will the acquired inpatient
  business bring new outpatient business as well?
  Because the buyer in this case has excess inpatient capacity but not outpatient capacity, it
  would have to expand outpatient facilities to accommodate the incremental outpatient volumes.
  This additional business also creates incremental
  working capital needs for the buyer.

- *Legal requirements.* In the state in which the hospitals are located, the buyer must obtain a certifi-
  cate of need to move the inpatient beds. The state
  further requires that a facility must remain open
  at least 12 months after announcing its closure.
  The latter legal requirement creates additional
  and significant capital expenditures and ongoing
  operating needs at the seller facility.

Clearly, these issues—especially the question of
medical staff loyalty, the need to invest in outpatient
facilities, and the state's intimidating legal requirements—weigh heavily in the buyer's decision. The
need to translate these uncertainties into hard numbers is clear.

Approach

The buyer's approach in this case is incremental. The
acquisition analysis first will test the buyer's ability to
absorb the seller's utilization by closing the seller's
facility and calculating the value of that incremental

business. Eventually, we will estimate the value of the facility's future alternative uses, although this should not and will not enhance the price the purchaser would be willing to pay, since these alternative uses do not actually provide existing business and cash flow. The heart of the analysis, though, is quite similar to the buy-and-operate scenario, as shown below:

- Define the incremental net income and cash flows that the acquired patient volumes will add to the buyer's baseline business.

- Determine vulnerable variables and perform sensitivity analyses to define a range of risk-adjusted incremental cash flows.

- Using the discounted cash flows, calculate the range of values for the incremental business.

These analyses must be based on the payer mix of the seller and the cost data of the buyer. The acquired patients will retain their payer mix, but the buyer must absorb them into its own revenue and cost base.

Valuation Analysis

To prepare the financial model for the valuation analysis, the buyer must:

- Develop a baseline revenue-and-expense model for its own operations.

- Get as much utilization-by-payer data as possible for the seller's patients.

- Pay close attention to fixed and variable expense assumptions at the buyer's facility, since they will be important in the incremental analysis.

- Model the incremental inpatient and outpatient business from the seller's facility and its effect on the existing operations of the buyer.

With these preparations made, the analyst subtracts the buyer's baseline financial forecasts from those forecasts prepared, including the business acquired from the seller. This provides the incremental cash flows generated by acquired business. Similar to the buy-and-operate scenario, the buyer selects the vulnerable variable(s) and calculates a range of discounted cash flows. Note that the discount rates used to calculate the net present value (NPV) of cash flows are higher in this scenario (15 and 18 percent) than in the first scenario (12.7 and 14.5 percent). The reason is that the perceived risk of this acquisition, given its dependence on an uncontrollable variable such as physician loyalty, is much higher.

Table 4-5 shows the range of cash flows incremental to this acquisition, adjusted for various buyer expectations for admissions volumes (low and high), discount rates (15 and 18 percent), and capital expenditure needs (none or $4 million to add outpatient facilities). The table further demonstrates the break-even point for the buyer, assuming a purchase price of $20 million. If, for example, the buyer made the $4 million investment in outpatient facilities and the discount rate was 15 percent, the average benefit to the buyer would be only $3.3 million. This information is

Table 4-5 Buy and Close: Net Present Value of Cash Flows Incremental to an Acquisition ($000s)

	Low Volume (1,776 admissions)		High Volume (1,942 admissions)			Average	
	15%	18%	15%	18%	Overall	15%	18%
No additional buyer capital expenditures	$24,763	$18,616	$29,850	$22,834	$24,016	$27,306	$20,725
$4 million capital expenditures	$20,763	$14,616	$25,850	$18,834	$20,016	$23,306	$16,725

Value Received Assuming a $20 Million Purchase Price

	Low Volume (1,776 admissions)		High Volume (1,942 admissions)			Average	
	15%	18%	15%	18%	Overall	15%	18%
No additional buyer capital expenditures	$4,763	($1,384)	$9,850	$2,834	$4,016	$7,306	$725
$4 million capital expenditures	$763	($5,384)	$5,850	($1,166)	$16	$3,306	($3,275)

charted in Figure 4-1 to emphasize the operating performance levels the buyer would need to attain just to
break even.

Results

Convinced by the analytic evidence, the hospital decides not to acquire its nearby competitor. The success
of the acquisition, planners decide, is too dependent
on physician loyalty. The 1,600 incremental admissions necessary to break even on a $20 million invest-
ment is likely unachievable.

Furthermore, the intended alternative uses of the
closed institution are not properly suited to its acute
care facility. Any conversion would require public ap-
provals, and the new psychiatric, rehabilitation, or

**Figure 4-1 Buy and Close: Showing Value Received
Assuming a $20 Million Purchase Price**

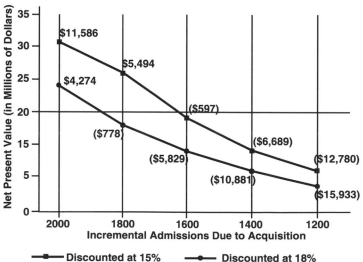

skilled nursing services would require the buyer to establish entirely new patient markets.

In short, the acquisition analysis has convinced the hospital that its $20 million would be better spent on recapturing and then increasing its local market share for existing business.

A Case Study: Buy and Reconfigure

A 150-bed rural acute care hospital's only direct competitor is a 55-bed, for-profit, and mostly private-pay hospital on the other side of town. The larger institution, part of a regional system, has attracted all but a few physicians away from the smaller hospital and now needs room to expand to accommodate increasing utilization. In an attempt to recapture utilization, the smaller hospital is constructing a wing to expand its surgery department.

A private developer has offered to buy the smaller hospital and lease it back to the larger hospital. In effect, the developer has interrupted the slow absorption of the smaller hospital into the larger institution and forced the larger hospital into a decision. The larger hospital's planners must decide whether it makes more sense to wait patiently for the smaller hospital to close or to move now, acquiring both the private-pay admissions and a facility to house expanding operations. Then, if acquisition is deemed the prudent course, should the hospital lease from the developer or buy the facility itself?

Issues to Consider

The buy-and-reconfigure scenario is essentially an organizational merger. Because the facilities must be converted to accommodate shared services and staff, physical renovations at both facilities will require capital expenditures. There are several other important issues for the buyer to consider here:

- *Admissions and medical staff.* With so few physicians and patients left at the smaller hospital, what real value do they hold? In this case, the seller's medical staff was refused privileges at the buyer's institution, so the physicians are actually considered a liability in the sale. The private payer mix of their admissions, however, is attractive.

- *Economies of scale.* The reconfiguration would require additional staffing for the transportation of materials and patients between the two facilities.

- *Community response.* The community is uneasy with the prospect of becoming a one-hospital town.

In addition to these factors, the seller's year-to-date financial performance shows a rapid deterioration.

Approach

The analytic approach here is much the same as in the buy-and-close scenario. The incremental analysis in this case, however, must incorporate the costs to keep the seller's facility operating. As the analysis evolves, though, the real choice the buyer faces is whether to go ahead and reconfigure the merged institution or, instead, close the acquired facility outright. In addition, the buyer is gaining more and more of the seller's patients due to medical staff unrest. Table 4-6 shows the results of the acquisition analysis comparing the conversion and closure scenarios in terms of average daily census, incremental cash flows, the buyer's additional capital expenditures, and the cash flow required to fund the purchase. With this table, the buyer and its parent system could evaluate at a glance the facility's present value and break-even value under each scenario.

Results

Clearly, closing the seller's facility provides the greatest economic benefit to the buyer. At an incremental average daily census of 15, the break-even value of that business is almost $13.5 million. Considering the seller's rapidly declining utilization, however, the acquisition becomes less attractive to the buyer. The seller's financial predicament looks bleaker with every month, and physician departures from the smaller hospital are on the rise. By the time the buyer and representatives of its parent system meet, the expected incremental census to the buyer drops by half to only seven. The buyer and its parent system decide to make an offer of $3 million, a number chosen informally, based on four incremental patients per day, to get negotiations started.

The seller refuses the offer. As in the previous case studies, the seller adheres to a sales price of six times

Table 4-6   Buy and Reconfigure: Present Value Cash Flow Evaluations of the Proposed Acquisition

(amounts in $000s)	Projections						Purchase Price $9,000 Discount Rate 14.00%
	1993	1994	1995	1996	1997	1998 and Beyond	Present Value of Cash Flows
Buyer Baseline	$962	$1,277	$1,408	$1,349	$1,197		
Close Seller							
Average Daily Census of 15							
Incremental Cash Flow	$1,242	$2,150	$2,326	$2,496	$2,668	$19,055	$15,858
Add'l Capital Expenditures at Buyer	(2,380)						(2,380)
Cash Flow to Fund Purchase	(9,000)						(9,000)
Present Value to System							$4,478
Break-even Value of Scenario $13,478							
Average Daily Census of 22							
Incremental Cash Flow	$1,617	$2,955	$3,174	$3,391	$3,608	$25,771	$21,457
Add'l Capital Expenditures at Buyer	(2,380)						(2,380)
Cash Flow to Fund Purchase	(9,000)						(9,000)
Present Value to System							$10,077
Break-even Value of Scenario $19,077							

Continued on next page

Table 4-6 Buy and Reconfigure: Present Value Cash Flow Evaluations of the Proposed Acquisition (continued)

(amounts in $000s)	Projections					1998 and Beyond	Present Value of Cash Flows
	1993	1994	1995	1996	1997		
					Purchase Price $9,000		
					Discount Rate 14.00%		
Buyer Baseline	$962	$1,277	$1,408	$1,349	$1,197		
Close Seller							
Average Daily Census of 15							
Incremental Cash Flow	$780	$1,599	$1,710	$1,795	$1,878	$13,416	$11,219
Add'l Capital Expenditures at Buyer	(2,380)	(621)	(655)	(610)	(500)	($3,571)	(5,999)
Cash Flow to Fund Purchase	(9,000)						(9,000)
Present Value to System							($3,780)
Break-even Value of Scenario $5,220							
Average Daily Census of 22							
Incremental Cash Flow	$1,154	$2,404	$2,558	$2,691	$2,819	$20,132	$16,818
Add'l Capital Expenditures at Buyer	(2,380)	(621)	(665)	(610)	(500)	($3,571)	(5,999)
Cash Flow to Fund Purchase	(9,000)						(9,000)
Present Value to System							$1,819
Break-even Value of Scenario $10,819							

* Cash flows are converted to present values using a 14% discount rate.
* The "1998 & Beyond" column shows the discounted value of the 1997 cash flow continuing in perpetuity.

the previous year's cash flow. Furthermore, it maintains that the medical staff will soon return to the facility and improve overall utilization. Today, however, the larger facility continues to erode the smaller hospital's market at a steady pace.

Conclusion

All three of the acquisition scenarios presented in this chapter can be counted as successes for the buyer or potential buyer. Through skillful financial analysis, each was able to fully inform its decisionmakers and carefully consider the strategic implications of the acquisition. Even the decision not to acquire, as in the buy-and-close and buy-and-reconfigure examples, leaves the financially capable healthcare organization in an excellent market position. In fact, the very process of analyzing an acquisition builds the buyer's knowledge of its local competitors, clarifies its own strategic options, and bolsters its financial advantage and preparedness for future struggles in the marketplace.

CHAPTER 5

Jason H. Sussman

Analysis and Sizing of Project Investments

The real power of financial planning is that the individual analyses build on one another. An organization can start with the financial planning exercise outlined in Chapter 2 to create a plan that will provide a basic financial roadmap. Quality financial decisionmaking, however, depends on the organization's ability to intensify the rigor of the analyses and to answer increasingly difficult questions. Is the organization allocating its resources toward appropriate investments? Are the dollars required appropriate given the expected returns? Is the scope of the proposed investment consistent with the organization's financial capabilities? The financial plan and its subsidiary analyses serve to align the organization's strategic, operating, and financial initiatives.

The most significant challenge to the organization's financial equilibrium is, of course, the large project. A project can be defined as "large" when its scope places an organization in a situation in which the project-related financial commitments could jeopardize the organization's financial flexibility, strain its operating capabilities, and interfere with its pursuit of a predetermined strategic vision.

To closely scrutinize the project-specific impact of a proposed investment, the financially capable organization shifts easily from the macroanalytical perspective provided by the financial and capital planning process to a more microanalytic technique. The skills employed to develop the overall financial framework provided by the financial planning process can readily be employed to analyze individual project investments as well.

In this chapter we introduce an effective analytic approach for assessing capital investments. Although useful for project investments of any size, this process is especially effective for evaluating projects that could threaten the financial integrity of the organization. Too often, development of an affordable project size and associated financing structure becomes an exercise characterized by elaborate guesswork. Worse, such guesswork is often laced with political input from managers with programmatic interests and from external players, either on the organization's board or parties potentially involved in the project's completion.

As demonstrated in the following case study, it is through careful analysis and thoughtful presentation of vital information that a management team can apply strict, objective mathematical logic to quantitatively determine the right investment amount for a project based on the organization's identified long-term financial goals. The situation described in this chapter not only illustrates a typical management interaction but also goes further in delineating an analytic process that led management, as a unified team, to return to its board of directors with a major capital project of significantly *reduced* size. In the end, the strategic intentions of the project were fully preserved, while the ability of the organization to assure its long-term financial competitiveness was retained and enhanced.

An Analytic Approach to Project Sizing

The analysis of an individual project investment depends on the strong foundation established by the financial and capital planning process. As delineated in Chapter 2, this process is the means by which the organization establishes and quantifies its key short- and long-term financial targets *and* the operational structure by which those targets will be achieved. The project analysis then weighs a particular proposed investment against the organization's broader strategic financial goals. The purpose of the analysis is to define an appropriate project investment given the organization's financial targets, planned strategic initiatives, and resulting achievable operating levels. This is a delicate balance achieved by all financially successful organizations.

Project investment analysis and sizing is a natural extension of the financial planning process. The basic modeling techniques employed are similar but are modified to focus more specifically on the long-term effects of a particular project investment. Beginning with a projection of the organization's operations under a "business-as-usual" scenario, the projection scenarios are further refined to include various strategic initiatives and alternative capital investment levels. With the use of the organization's long-term financial objectives as a point of reference, assessment of the costs and benefits of specific capital investments is straightforward.

Implicit in the project sizing process is the need to implement a rigorous, methodical approach to the ultimate sizing of a specific capital project. This process includes the following general steps:

1. *Organizational financial targets.* The establishment of appropriate long-term organizational financial goals consistent with performance levels required to access the capital markets creates the basic framework for all levels of financial analysis. Review and understanding of financial performance levels of peer institutions (especially in terms of the organization's desired level of creditworthiness) provides a valid means to measure ongoing organizational performance as well as the appropriateness of proposed capital investments.

The analysis of a project investment is valid only if a meaningful context is established in which to perform the assessment. The financially competitive organization will have already created this context through periodic updates of its long-term financial and capital plan. For the organization that has not yet completed such a plan, project analysis must follow evaluation of the organization's financial position and establishment of realistic targets for financial performance.

The basis for this undertaking is the credit analysis. This analysis provides an indication of the trends over time and, in comparison to peer organizations, of an institution's financial performance. Through evaluation of specific financial ratios, management can evaluate its ongoing financial performance and ability to access capital. Remember from Chapter 2 that the credit analysis includes a limited number of ratios representing a small subset of the vast array of potential financial ratios which can be calculated. Once again, the suggested ratios include:

- Debt service coverage
- Operating margin
- Excess margin
- Capitalization ratio
- Cushion ratio
- Days cash on hand
- Days in accounts receivable
- Average age of plant

These basic ratios provide significant insight into the financial performance of any organization and are the computational building blocks for many other ratios often cited. Furthermore, these ratios interact in such a way as to provide the analyst with an enhanced understanding of the financial dynamics of the organization and the relationship of such historical financial performance to the subset of proposed investments.

2. *Organizational capital position.* Ongoing profitability or, more correctly, cash flow requirements must be quantified to support outcome measurement. By understanding the magnitude of the difference between the organization's currently available capital and its requirements for funding principal payments, capital investment needs, and balance sheet reserves, management actually can calculate specific annual cash flow targets for performance at varying levels of capital investment, given specific investment decisions.

The capital position analysis provides a means to communicate the magnitude of an organization's need to generate ongoing operating cash flows. This analysis hinges on the financial targets established in step 1 and the level of *total* capital investment proposed by the organization. (Again, as noted in Chapter 2, the capital position analysis illustrates the relationship of the organization's sources of capital to its proposed uses of capital.)

3. *Organizational operating projections.* Understanding the practical financial capabilities of an organization requires an in-depth awareness of the key business levers that impact operating results. Through a structured process of projection development and refinement, management can determine not only the organization's potential for cash flow generation, but also the key operational areas of management concern on which such cash generation will be dependent. The process of refining the projections also underscores the integral link between operating requirements and the timing and total amount of capital expenditures.

4. *Project sizing and financing structure.* Comparison of the projected financial results to the organization's established financial targets provides a means by which to quantify the maximum supportable project investment. Furthermore, when management is armed with an awareness of the interaction of the various financial target requirements, the optimal debt and equity investment mix for the project can be set mathematically.

5. *Risk assessment.* As much as management often likes to believe it is able to predict a "most likely" operating scenario, actual results *never* fully meet expectations. Therefore, perhaps the most important step of the project sizing analysis is assessing the ability of the organization to continue to support a defined project investment

under a wide range of potential operating assumptions. This risk assessment serves two purposes. First, it establishes the level of risk associated with an amount of project investment. Management and the board can decide whether such risk is excessive. Second, through evaluation of the incremental impact of changes in various assumptions, management is able to focus resources on operating areas that most affect project investment outcomes.

Although the project sizing process described in steps 1 through 5 is structured to be objective and logical, the entire investment analysis is founded on a set of assumptions of future business conditions developed by management. Chances are that perhaps one in three of those assumptions will ultimately reflect reality. Therefore, it is vital that the uncertainty and resulting impact related to the underlying assumptions be fully exposed and evaluated.

To a large extent, these steps mirror the more standard financial and capital planning process. However, the serious potential financial implications of a significant project investment require intensified rigor and discipline. The financially capable healthcare organization is prepared to launch such project analysis at a moment's notice because this analytic process is a basic staple of institutionalized financial decisionmaking. Many organizations attempt project-specific analyses without the support of a formal financial planning process. These attempts are intellectually and mathematically backward and often lead to inappropriate and illogical conclusions. The following case study demonstrates the foundation and context provided by the financial plan and the investment analyses that are easily and explicitly drawn from the larger context.

A Case Study: Project Sizing

A new CFO has joined a large hospital, Regional Medical Center, which has just completed a long, complex, and politically taxing strategic master planning process for its facility. An important recommendation of the resulting plan includes a major facility renovation and expansion project. The facility master plan, budgeted at $33.2 million, calls for the replacement of inpatient and intensive care unit beds and the expansion of certain ambulatory care areas on the main campus of the acute care facility. Based on an initial review, the CFO has significant concerns regarding the magnitude of the project investment. The CFO fears that the proposed level of capital investment might threaten Regional Medical Center's long-term financial position. This is based, in part, on a broad-based debt capacity analysis prepared for the medical center by an investment banker who hopes to underwrite the financing associated with the project. Even though this analysis shows significant available debt capacity, the CFO is not satisfied.

Unable to quantify and properly communicate intuitive concerns about the proposed project, the CFO begins development of a comprehensive strategic financial plan for the medical center as a first step in an in-depth review of the long-term financial consequences of the facility master plan. The goal of this financial planning process is *not* to cajole the CEO and other key managers into reconsidering the relative strategic importance of the project—the strategic issues are a given. Rather, by modifying and augmenting analyses that are basic to corporate finance-based financial planning, the CFO seeks to specify a level of capital investment and to quantify a project investment that is appropriately matched with objective financial targets and achievable operating results. The basic steps implemented at Regional Medical Center illustrate an analytic framework for assessing any capital investment, as described below.

Step 1: Organizational Financial Targets

The credit analysis for Regional Medical Center, shown in Table 5-1, describes a picture of financial stability and strength. The medical center's operating margin has increased steadily, and its excess (profit) margin remains consistent. Debt service coverage also has been consistent at relatively high levels.

The weakest aspect of the medical center's financial structure, reflected by its capitalization ratio, is its high leverage position. The Regional's capital structure, however, includes $30 million of variable rate debt. When the variable rate 1991 bonds are excluded from calculation of the capitalization ratio, Regional Medical Center's leverage is reduced to acceptable levels. Conversely, the real *strength* of the medical center is its cash position, with "days cash on hand" consistently in excess of 100 days. It is this strength, how-

Table 5-1 Credit Analysis Highlights

Ratio	1992 S&P "A" Rated Hospitals	1992 Moody's "A" Rated Hospitals	Regional Medical Center		
			1991	1992	Projected 1993
Debt Service Coverage	3.0x	3.1x	3.4x	3.7x	3.7x
Operating Margin	4.8%	3.4%	1.7%	4.0%	4.4%
Excess Margin	6.6%	5.4%	4.1%	5.9%	4.8%
Debt/Capitalization	32.3%	42.2%	49.5%	47.9%	45.3%
Debt/Capitalization (without 1991 debt)	32.3%	42.2%	32.8%	31.2%	28.8%
Cushion Ratio	6.1x	5.7x	9.0x	6.9x	7.0x
Days Cash on Hand	141.0 days	98.2 days	145.2 days	127.9 days	123.3 days
Days in Accts. Rec. (Net)	68.5 days	70.0 days	74.1 days	77.0 days	76.2 days
Average Age of Plant	7.4 years	7.6 years	8.1 years	8.5 years	9.0 years

ever, that is also a "red flag" in this credit analysis. Over the last three years, the medical center has seen a decline in "days cash on hand" while at the same time its average age of plant has increased. (This increase is, in fact, the strategic basis for the proposed facility plan.) Therefore, even though the medical center has not invested excessive amounts of capital or supported abnormal working capital requirements (e.g., accounts receivable) over the evaluation period, it has still seen some deterioration in its cash position. Although the projected 1993 cash levels are by no means at a critical stage, the deterioration of the medical center's cash position highlights the need to evaluate alternative sources of funds to finance the proposed facility plan.

Much can be learned from this chronological credit analysis, but it is vital to extend the credit analysis and compare the organization's performance to an appropriate peer group.

The CFO's initial evaluation of Regional Medical Center's financial performance leads to the selection of the universe of "A" rated hospitals as an appropriate peer group. Review of the medical center's historical performance indicates that this choice is perhaps conservative; a more aggressive approach would challenge the medical center to match the financial performance of the next higher credit rating, an "A+" rating. The medical center's performance has exceeded or been consistent with "A" rated median levels for each of the past three years.

In short, the credit analysis indicates that Regional Medical Center is in step with its peers. To maintain that financial competitiveness, the medical center must somehow lower its average age of plant without depleting its cash reserves. These findings provide a solid beginning for the CFO to communicate the previously stated concerns regarding the size of the proposed facility plan. The credit analysis creates an objective context by which the organization can judge the medical center's financial performance and establish objective long-term financial goals. A table such as Table 5-1 is especially useful in communicating this vital information to the organization's nonfinancial management.

Given acceptance of "A" rated performance as Regional Medical Center's financial objective, the CFO then uses the associated medians to establish specific financial performance targets, as shown in Table 5-2.

The focus of these financial objectives is to enhance liquidity and minimize overall leverage, the most significant credit issues facing the medical center. The CFO assumes that current levels of profitability will set a minimum performance standard.

Table 5-2 Financial Performance Targets

Key Ratios	Pro Forma Targets
Target Debt Service Coverage	≥ 3.0 times
Maximum Capitalization Ratio	$\leq 50\%$
Target Capitalization Ratio	$\leq 32.3\%$
Minimum Days Cash on Hand	≥ 100 days
Target Days Cash on Hand	≥ 140 days

Step 2: Organizational Capital Position

Prior planning processes at Regional Medical Center had focused solely on the facility project investment of $33.2 million and ignored $38.3 million of additional capital requirements associated with routine equipment replacement and renovation. Ignoring routine capital replacement leads the CEO and other management team members to overrate the medical center's ability to make capital investments. Upon recognition of this vulnerability, the management team becomes more interested in calculating the medical center's ability to support all its planned capital requirements but especially the proposed facility improvements project.

As indicated in Tables 5-3 and 5-4, given the anticipated capital investment levels of Regional Medical Center, future operations (from 1994 to 1998) must generate at least $79.8 million of cash flow to enable the medical center to make its planned capital investments and retain a strong balance sheet. On average, this level of cash flow will require improvement of almost $5 million over current-year cash flow levels (see Table 5-4). This mathematical analysis puts the situation in perspective; the organization must enjoy improved profitability to generate the level of capital consistent with investment of approximately $71.5 million over the next five years. In a straightforward and nonjudgmental manner, the CFO has communicated the integral relationships between operating results and capital investment to the rest of the management team.

Table 5-3   Capital Position Analysis, 1994-98

Uses		
Recurring Needs, 1994-98	$38,300	
Facility Master Plan	33,225	
Total Asset Acquisition, 1994-98		$71,525
Funding of Minimum Cash Position		
(140 days of 1998 operating expenses)		43,362
Principal Payments on Existing Debt, 1994-98		3,800
Total Capital Uses		**$118,687**
Sources		
Existing Cash (1993 Cash and Marketable		
Securities and Board Designated Assets)		$31,100
Total 1993 Debt Capacity	$68,404	
Less: Total Debt Outstanding	(58,690)	
Less: Approximate Nonproject Proceeds	(1,943)	
Net Available Debt Capacity		7,771
Total Capital Sources		**$38,871**
Five-Year Cash Flow Requirement		**$79,816**

The immediate reaction of the nonfinancial managers is to eliminate, defer, or downsize the project. While one of these responses is likely to be a part of the medical center's ultimate financial/operating plan, the CFO defers a decision pending further

Table 5-4   Capital Allocation Summary of Overall Profitability Requirements ($000s)

	Cash Flow	Cash Margin
Five-Year Cash Flow Requirement	$79,816	$79,816
Projected Total Operating and		
Nonoperating Revenue	xxxxxx	$604,993
Required Average to Meet Capital	$15,963	13.2%
Needs		
1993 Projected Level	$11,058	10.6%
1992 Actual Level	$11,335	11.7%

analysis to increase management's understanding of specifically how project size has an impact on operating requirements.

Step 3: Organizational Financial Projections

The CFO determines that, given the management culture at Regional Medical Center, the best way to evaluate the true impact of the project will be to focus on a "business-as-usual" approach to fund only routine capital expenditures, thereby isolating the $33 million capital investment for later consideration.

To create business-as-usual projections, assumptions are developed and reviewed with the CEO, COO, and other key management members. In that way, the projections belong to management, not just the CFO, and any conclusions associated with the projection will be received more openly.

The major objectives of this step are to:

- Project Regional Medical Center's financial performance without implementation of the facility master plan.

- Revise the operating projections to reflect any market strategies that will be undertaken to preserve volumes and revenue as well as any operating strategies, such as expense and financial controls, that will be put in place.

- Compare those revised baseline projections with the established financial targets.

Table 5-5 shows the results of this business-as-usual scenario. Regional Medical Center's projected financial performance—incorporating certain key contemplated market and operating strategies but disregarding the facility renovation—easily meets or exceeds every financial target. Therefore, the baseline operating results do indeed support the organization's routine capital needs. But how will these baseline projections be affected by various levels of debt financing required to support the facility master plan?

Table 5-5 Partial Analysis Comparison of Baseline Results to Targets ($000s)

	Baseline Projected 1998	Financial Targets
Net Income	$10,723	$8,878
Unrestricted Cash	$70,823	$43,362
Net Revenue Margin	5.3%	N/A
Debt Service Coverage	6.1×	3.0×
Capitalization Ratio	33.2%	32.3%
Cushion Ratio	17.6×	6.1×
Days Cash on Hand	228.7 days	140 days
Excess Cash Margin	15.9%	12.4%

Step 4: Project Sizing and Financial Structure

Isolating the proposed project from the operating projections in step 3 establishes a performance baseline against which Regional Medical Center can measure the effect of the capital project. In step 4, the project is returned to the analysis through an iterative process that determines an appropriate project size based on the organization's operating capabilities and financing considerations. The calculations, which entail solving simultaneous equations, are complex and therefore require rather sophisticated financial modeling capabilities. The outcomes derived, however, are strictly mathematical and are easily understood.

The objective of this step is to quantify a project size and related level of debt financing that the medical center can support without jeopardizing its financial competitiveness. It is essential to follow a stepwise approach to project sizing, taking the time to observe the effects of each variable and to test the results against financial targets.

Table 5-6 reflects the result of the first phase of the project sizing analysis. This table compares the end-point (i.e., 1998) financial results generated, assuming investment of $33.2 million in the facility plan project using two purely arbitrary debt levels. This initial analysis indicates the following:

- Either level of debt, $25 or $30 million, will increase Regional Medical Center's capitalization ratio to levels in excess of the 50 percent maximum established as an organizational financial target.

- The equity contribution required to fund the project using only $25 million of debt would reduce the medical center's cash levels during the projection period well below its 100-day minimum. Cash levels in 1998, however, are projected to exceed the 140-day target.

- The combination of debt and equity exceeds the actual project amount. This is because the pro-

Table 5-6   Impact of Debt Financing on 1998 Financial Results Assuming a $33.2 Million Project Cost ($000s)

	Financial Targets	Baseline Projection	Debt Scenarios	
			$25 Million	$30 Million
Equity Contribution Required	N/A	N/A	$12,300	$8,250
1998 Debt Service Coverage	3.0×	6.1×	4.0×	3.8×
1998 Operating Income	$6,263	$6,694	$3,701	$3,398
1998 Net Revenue Margin	N/A	5.3%	3.0%	2.7%
1998 Unrestricted Cash	$43,362	$70,823	$48,373	$52,475
Maximum Capitalization	≈50.0%	43.3%	52.4%	53.8%
1998 Capitalization	32.3%	33.2%	44.7%	46.1%
Minimum Days of Cash	100 Days	134 Days	85 Days	101 Days
1998 Cash	140 Days	229 Days	154 Days	167 Days

ceeds are also funding associated financing costs such as capitalized interest, debt service reserve fund, and issuance expenses. These financing costs vary directly with debt amount and indirectly with equity contribution.

The aspect of the analysis that complicates the financial decisionmaking process is the projection of strong financial results by 1998. A decision to pursue the $33.2 million project could be supported if all of management's expectations are achieved. However, during the initial two to three years of project development, the medical center's financial strength will be jeopardized, severely limiting the organization' strategic flexibility. After lengthy discussion among the key members of management representing all functional areas of the medical center, it is determined that the highly competitive nature of the hospital's market requires a plan that will maximize the medical center's long-term financial flexibility.

To quantify such flexibility, the CFO returns to the initial financial targets for capitalization and cash levels as benchmarks against which to calculate an appropriate project size. The approach answers the following questions:

- What is the maximum equity contribution that the medical center can make to the project and still retain the minimum level of cash of 100 days?

- What is the maximum amount of new debt that the medical center can issue and remain at or below 50 percent capitalization?

- Given levels of debt and equity, and current capital markets conditions regarding interest rates and amortization, what is the maximum supportable project investment?

Table 5-7 quantifies the answers to these questions. The analysis indicates that, given the above constraints, Regional Medical Center's maximum debt and equity to support the project are $17.3 million and $8.5 million, respectively. Factoring these maxima into the sources and uses equation delineated in Table 5-7, a maximum project size of $22.8 million is calculated.

The analysis results in an appropriate project size almost $10 million less than the project defined in the facility master plan. Clearly, management is not thrilled with the prospect of reworking the project to fit the new dollar parameter, nor does it look forward to returning to the board to say, "We made a mistake." The logic of the process is, however, inescapable.

Table 5-7   Total Project Cost Calculated to Meet Target Financial Measures

Uses	
Facility Master Plan Costs	$22,800
Capitalized Interest	2,074
Debt Service Reserve Fund	1,289
Underwriter's Discount	156
Other Issuance Costs	500
Total Project	**$26,819**

Sources	
Debt Proceeds	$17,284
Equity Contribution	8,500
Interest During Construction	1,035
Total Project	**$26,819**

As indicated in Table 5-8, the financial results associated with the revised project investments are projected to meet every financial target established. (The only exception is target capitalization, which declines only to 41.3 percent, above the target of 32.3 percent.

Step 5: Risk Assessment

Because of the number of assumptions used to generate the financial projections, presentation and analysis of all possible assumption permutations would, quite frankly, undo most of the benefits derived through the structure and efficiency of the preceding four steps. Therefore, it is incumbent on the person driving the process (the CFO at Regional Medical Center) to evaluate a variety of assumptions and identify those assumption changes that most materially impact the agreed-upon plan. For the medical center, those variables are identified and evaluated in Table 5-9.

The medical center's management spends a significant amount of time identifying and evaluating the key assumptions underlying the operating projections. The major areas include:

- *Volume*—Changes in overall admissions, general outpatient growth, and varying levels of activity of one of the medical center's key services, cardiac surgery.

- *Revenue*—Impact of rate increases and reimbursement rate changes.

Table 5-8 Impact on Projected Financial Position Assuming a $22.8 Million Facility Master Plan Cost (Total Project Cost of $26.8 Million) ($000s)

	Financial Targets	Baseline Results	Reduced Project $17.3 Million Debt
Equity Contribution Required	N/A	N/A	$8,500
1998 Debt Service Coverage	3.0×	6.1×	4.5×
1998 Operating Income	$6,408	$6,694	$4,628
1998 Net Revenue Margin	N/A	5.3%	3.7%
1998 Unrestricted Cash	$43,918	$70,823	$55,310
Maximum Capitalization	≈50.0%	43.3%	49.9%
1998 Capitalization	32.3%	33.2%	41.3%
Minimum Days of Cash	100 Days	134 Days	100 Days
1998 Cash	140 Days	229 Days	177 Days

Table 5-9   Estimated Impact of Risk Scenarios

	Impact on 1998 Operating Income	Impact on 1998 Cash Position	Impact on 1998 Net Revenue Margin
Baseline Results with Recommended Project Size	$4,628	177.0 Days	3.7%
Risk Scenarios:			
Favorable			
1. Flat Admissions	$135	0 Days	0.1%
2. Cardiac Surgery Growth	$1,600	17 Days	1.3%
3. Fund Raising	0	31 Days	0.0%
4. Increase Medicare Case Mix Index	$1,425	16 Days	1.1%
Unfavorable			
5. Lower Price Increases	($980)	(12 Days)	(0.8%)
6. Reduced Outpatient Growth	($1,490)	(10 Days)	(1.2%)
7. No Productivity	($1,400)	(13 Days)	(1.1%)
8. Increased HMO/PPO Discounts	($1,580)	(13 Days)	(1.3%)

- *Expenses*—Key staffing assumptions as a challenge to management's ability to accomplish the full-time equivalent (FTE) staff reductions assumed.

Each risk scenario is compared to the baseline operating results for 1998. For example, if management were not able to achieve productivity enhancement as assumed (see risk scenario 7 in Table 5-9), 1998 operating income would be reduced by $1.4 million and days cash would also be reduced by 13 days. As a result, 1998 operating income would be $3,268,000, and the medical center would have 164 days of cash on hand. While this is a material impact, the resulting levels of financial performance are such that the project investment could still be sustained.

This conclusion is the same for each risk scenario tested. Furthermore, management believes that it has the ability and flexibility to control operations under any of the risk scenarios presented. Therefore, management was able to develop a strong sense of comfort as to the appropriateness of the revised project investment.

The risk assessment serves two purposes. First and foremost, it clarifies the risk levels associated with the facility master plan. That is, it answers the questions, How successful does management need to be in achieving its operating goals to make the project work? and What would the nature of management's responses need to be under varying operating conditions? The responses to these questions provide management and the board with a more complete understanding of the ongoing operating risks associated with a given capital investment.

The second purpose of the risk assessment is to support the allocation of management resources. Armed with a knowledge of the key success variables for the organization (they are different for every organization), management can allocate time and resources to those areas. Through active monitoring of these key areas and knowing the actual results required for success, management is positioned to proactively adjust operations to changes in the identified key variables.

Results

At Regional Medical Center, management presents the CFO's analysis, unchanged, to a special joint meeting of the planning and finance committees and to the board as a whole. Management is pleasantly surprised by the board's reaction to this apparently "revisionist analysis." The board feels that, for the first time, governance has an understanding of the comprehensive financial impact of the project on the medical center. Furthermore, the board is convinced that the revised project budget is consistent with maintaining the fiscal integrity of Regional Medical Center yet still will be sufficient to accomplish the master plan's strategic intent.

By applying analytic skills to the issue at hand, the CFO has translated intuitive concerns into quantified, logical findings and has communicated those findings in a convincing, straightforward manner. The results of the process validate the CFO's concerns and, most importantly, provide a means by which those concerns can be communicated to the rest of management in a highly objective, analytic format. At the same time, development of the long-term strategic financial plan provides a useful organizational bonus. Year one of that plan will be Regional Medical Center's budget framework for 1994. Most importantly, through institutionalization of the financial planning process, the CFO insures a continued ability to include finance in the medical center's strategic decisionmaking process.

Conclusion

Successful project analysis requires a testing of the true impact of an individual project investment, tailoring the investment to best reflect the organization's operating realities and better serve its long-term strategic vision. But project analysis is only a tool, and tools must be skillfully applied to be effective.

Bringing all of the decisionmaking discipline and analytic rigor of the financial planning process to bear on a single capital investment is a clear object lesson in financial planning. Any healthcare organization contemplating a major capital project will find that the capability and analytic resources required to perform such an analysis are no longer luxuries of large institutions with large financial staffs. The increased risks associated with more competitive and dynamic markets mandate that management implement any and all processes that can minimize decisionmaking errors or, at least, reduce the financial impact of such errors. The financial planning process, along with the related investment-specific analyses described here are among the most vital and beneficial tools available to the healthcare executive. To include finance in strategic decisionmaking is perhaps the key accomplishment in creating a financially capable and competitive organization.

CHAPTER 6

Mark L. Hall and
Catherine E. Kleinmuntz

Physician-Hospital Integration Analysis

It is the rare hospital these days that does not have some physician-hospital integration activities underway. In some markets, the primary consideration may be the transition of solo practitioners to more efficient group practices. For other organizations, the focus may be on the development of a vehicle for better coordination of managed care issues or facilitation of the growth and development of existing physician groups. The important thing to recognize is that virtually all of these activities culminate in a transaction of some form and that the transaction is not a one-time occurrence but the formalization of a business relationship that is meant to last.

The recent popularity of seminars on this subject reflects an understanding that these activities involve complex issues of strategy, organization, politics, and finance while at the same time are fraught with numerous legal perils. Underlying this is a powerful sense of urgency created by continued development of managed care products and by interhospital competition to secure relationships with the most desirable physicians.

One common response to this sense of urgency is to attack all of the above-mentioned development issues in a single frenzied effort involving consultants, lawyers, and accountants. Sometimes this is due to an unexpected opportunity. In other cases, there is simply an attitude among certain individuals that the deal needs to get done, that careful analysis is nothing more than an impediment, and that the sooner the transaction is reduced to an organizational chart and set of legal documents, the better.

There are a number of risks inherent in pursuing these transactions in this manner. The most significant risk is a potential loss of perspective and the squandering of the organization's political and/or financial capital on the first deal. In moving too hastily, organizations fail to give themselves and the physicians an opportunity to truly understand the structural and financial dynamics of the transaction at hand.

The central theme of this chapter is that any physician-hospital integration project needs to be managed in the context of an orderly process, which is supported by rigorous financial analysis. Although it is certainly possible, and in some cases necessary, to tackle some of these steps out of sequence, it has been our experience that the most productive and stable transactions come as a result of careful planning and involvement. The technical analysis needs to be supported by attention to the organizational dynamics of the situation and to the decisionmaking processes to be used by each party. In this chapter, we will consider the process both in the abstract and in its application to a specific case.

The Process of Physician-Hospital Integration

Much has been made of the special nature of the activities of physician-hospital integration. However, it is our opinion that many of the philosophies and techniques described earlier in this book may be applied to physician-hospital integration via a five-step process, as follows:

1. Understand the strategic context.

2. Develop the business plan and understand the macroeconomics of the transaction.

3. Define the transaction.

4. Understand the microeconomics of the transaction.

5. Value the transaction.

These steps are discussed in detail below.

Step One: Understand the Strategic Context

This is not a book about strategy, but it is important to note that effective transaction development requires a strategic context that the principals understand well. It is surprising how many transactions proceed without this understanding. If nothing else, your investment in professional fees will be more efficient if you can provide those charged with structuring the transaction with some guidance and insight into the following:

1. *Market climate.* What is driving the integration urge at this time? Is capitation here, or is it a couple of years off? Is the strategy defensive or offensive?

2. *Physician climate.* A transaction requires at least two motivated parties. What is the level of urgency among the key physicians? What are their needs and barriers? What is the level of sophistication regarding the issues? Is more information required before embarking on a specific transaction? How are the local medical practices organized now? What would be an optimal organizational structure?

3. *Hospital climate.* The hospital needs to take stock of its own situation. It needs to consider its current market position and potential attraction to physician partners, the current state of relationships with the physicians, and the extent of the financial resources it can make available to fund

the strategy. The internal approval process needs to be constantly anticipated and managed.

4. *Development focus.* The integration strategy needs to provide specific direction related to targeted markets and/or payers as well as information on the required number and types of physicians and their geographic locations.

5. *Candidate assessment.* Any integration process has to start somewhere. The effective healthcare organization already will have decided its priorities. Some physician practices will represent an excellent base from which to begin, other practices will be better approached once some momentum toward integration has been established, and still others may have no place at all in the integration strategy. The ability of each group to support the development focus described above is a key consideration here.

Developing the above framework will require considerable analysis and thought, thus the most appropriate time to do this is when the organization is not distracted by the transaction implementation process.

Step Two: Develop the Business Plan and Understand the Macroeconomics of the Transaction

Having developed the strategic context and determined the best place to start, the next step is to develop a business vision and plan for the transaction at hand without regard (at this point) for legal structure and business terms. The plan should capture the

imagination of both parties and reinforce the basic
soundness of the relationship.

The hospital must answer two questions: (1) Assuming that we develop a relationship with this physician (or physician group), exactly what would we
try to do (e.g., operate as is, grow, add sites) and
(2) On what schedule would we like to do this? The
output of this analysis should be a business development narrative that is specific enough to identify capital requirements and develop financial projections.
Some executives believe that this step should take
place after the transaction has been put together
rather than before it. To us, this seems as futile as the
German shepherd who, after a lot of chasing, finally
sinks his teeth into a car's bumper—now what? In our
view, the process of developing a shared business vision will be a good test of the quality of the relationship.

The next task is to translate the business development narrative into a set of financial statements
driven by a specific set of planning assumptions. The
place to start is with an understanding of the operating economics of the existing practice(s). Do not un-
derestimate the amount of time it will take to develop
the data necessary to come to this understanding.
Usually, physician groups do not maintain the same
type of data bases that hospitals do. This does not
mean, however, that issues of utilization, payer mix,
productivity, and expense levels are not as critical to
the success of physicians as they are to that of hospitals. Stinting here in order to meet a hurry-up dead-
line virtually guarantees a breakdown later in the

process. The information infrastructure which is developed here will be the basis for measuring future success. The output at this stage should be a set of baseline financial projections for the medical practice under a set of status quo assumptions, which are not dissimilar to the baseline financial projections developed for the hospital in the financial planning process described in Chapter 2. Once the baseline is established, the model should be modified to reflect the initiatives identified in the business development narrative. This task provides an opportunity for the hospital to do some early due diligence on the physician practice. In many cases, the fundamental economics of the practice have turned out to be significantly different than what was thought at the outset of the analysis.

After the economic model is developed, it is necessary to assess the viability and the doability of the aggregate business plan. If the overall plan is unstable, no amount of creative transaction structuring can overcome such a fundamental flaw. The key points to consider in this assessment are:

- *Quality of results.* Does the aggregate enterprise generate sufficient cash flow to stay in business and provide a return on capital without regard to whose capital it is? Beware the transaction that is destined to become a financial black hole, regardless of whom may be footing the bill.

- *Affordability of growth.* Most physician-hospital integration plans contemplate growth in terms of physicians and/or sites. This growth necessitates cash for facilities and for working capital. The rate of growth can have a significant effect on the extent of the capital outlay. For example, in the case of a 30-physician group that was looking to expand to 150 physicians, the capital expense associated with achieving that growth in four years was more than twice that associated with pursuing that level of growth over a seven-year period because of the overlap of start-up costs. The hospital and the group simply did not have the funds to support a strategy based on the start-up of new practices. This resulted in a determination to focus attention on the addition of existing practices to the group.

- *Risk analysis.* It is important, if financial equilibrium is to be maintained, that all parties have a good grasp of the necessary trade-offs between the key variables. For example, in one situation it was determined that the three-physician site models that the physicians and hospital were considering to maximize geographic market share simply had too much start-up instability. For this reason, the emphasis was changed to fewer but potentially larger sites with a little less geographic coverage. In another situation, it was determined that the baseline finances could deteriorate rapidly and that a more aggressive development schedule was needed.

Based on the preceding three considerations, it is likely that the original business plan will be revised. It should reflect a framework that has a reasonable likelihood of success and that involves an acceptable level of expenditure and risk.

Step 3: Define the Transaction

If the parties involved have done adequate work up until now, everyone involved with the transaction should have a good understanding of the capital and organizational requirements associated with the business plan and with the aggregate financial dynamics of that plan. This, of course, assumes that the parties have been communicating openly throughout the analysis. As a result, the parties should be in a position to negotiate from a common understanding of the transaction at hand.

By now, the professionals charged with structuring the transaction should have enough information that they have some ideas as to what form the relationship should take and what transactions are necessary to implement that relationship. As a result, organizational charts and transaction flow exhibits should begin to surface. The questions to be addressed at this time are:

1. What will each negotiating party contribute to the business plan in terms of capital, operations, management, and governance?

2. What are the financial requirements associated with the above elements for each party?

3. How will the parties divide the revenues of the combined operations?

4. Who will own what?

5. What other terms and conditions are important?

Obviously, answering these questions is the most
sensitive part of the process since, in addition to basic
structure, the parties need to agree on who takes financial risk and how to divide the economic pie.
There is always a lot of give-and-take at this stage.
The working relationship, the shared vision, and the
basic understanding developed through the business
planning process should provide a base for arriving at
reasonable conclusions. The outcome of this portion
of the process should be a memorandum of understanding, which outlines the business terms and structure of the transaction.

Step 4: Understand the Microeconomics of the Transaction

Physician-hospital transactions need to last. To last,
they must be fair. Operationally this means that either
party should be willing to take either side of the deal.
One way to gauge the fairness of the transaction is to
understand its financial dynamics from both points of
view. To do this right requires that the financial analysis be refined to take into account the business plan
and the transaction definition as it has been developed thus far. The next step is to disaggregate the
business plan into its hospital and physician components.

Obviously, the first test for viability is whether each
component is financially stable under the accepted set

of business plan assumptions. The next level of analysis will determine whether underachievement or overachievement of the plan will unduly benefit or harm one of the parties or if variables under the control of one party can have substantial spillover effects on the other.

Based on the analysis, it may be necessary to reconfigure certain elements of the transaction in the interest of stability or fairness or both.

In one recent negotiation the preliminary transaction outline required the physicians to supervise and fund the start-up costs of new patient care personnel. The hospital was to handle the real estate and administrative requirements of the venture. The microlevel analysis identified the extent of the financial and management resources that would be required of the physicians. In this case, the decision was made to leave the transaction agreement as is, but it was important to all parties that the physicians gained a realistic assessment of their true financial exposure.

Step 5: Value the Transaction

A dilemma lies in answering a physician's question, How much are you willing to pay me for my practice? A wrong answer places a healthcare executive between the Scylla of potentially insulting a physician and losing him or her to a competitor and the Charybdis of creating an economically unstable transaction and/or violating the law. At this point, it becomes clear that the legal issues underlying fraud and abuse and tax-exempt status make these transactions extra difficult.

In the corporate world, transactions can be structured such that all parties can share significantly in the spillover effects resulting from the combination of their efforts. This is difficult to achieve in hospital-physician integration activities, since the most obvious spillover effects involve increased utilization at the hospital. On the other hand, many of the transactions closely resemble a venture capital model, in which the venture capitalist (hospital) is providing capital and additional management structure to the entrepreneur (physician) to help bring about more rapid and efficient entrepreneurial growth than would otherwise be the case. It is a rare venture capitalist who lets the entrepreneur take out a large sum of cash at the outset.

Still, the market will often dictate that the hospital make some payout to the physician. It is necessary that the payment be legal, sufficient, and economically supportable. It should be pointed out that, in many instances, these concepts have a high likelihood of being mutually exclusive, particularly if the subject of price is dealt with out of context.

The good news is that the laws and principles that govern these issues are becoming more explicit, making good legal work easier to understand. In many cases, an appraisal by an accounting firm is necessary. It is typically useful to have an upfront discussion of the appraisal methods used so that the business planning can be supportive to the process.

The issue of sufficiency from the point of view of the physicians will relate to the quality of the legal and accounting advice they are getting, their egos and expectations, the quality of the relationship with the hospital, and their view of what the relationship can provide them compared with other alternatives.

The concept of economic supportability requires a price and payout mechanism, which is affordable from the perspective of the hospital and sustainable in terms of the ongoing operations of the venture. It should reflect an application of the corporate finance principles described in Chapter 3.

This is obviously a critical point in the transaction development. The ability to move to closure requires a stable negotiating environment, which is best supported by thoughtful financial and legal analysis. Unfortunately, these processes do not guarantee success; random elements have a way of creating more turns and loops than anyone could imagine and there is still the likelihood that the whole effort could unravel on a moment's notice. Still, if you get past this point and agree on a business plan, structure, and terms, your chances of actually implementing the transaction are very high, and the care you have invested in the planning and development process will have paid off.

A Case Study: Physician-Hospital Integration

Community General Hospital is a 300-bed, not-for-profit hospital located in the suburbs of a major metropolitan area in the Southeast. The service area is

fairly competitive, with most of the competition still
focused on fee-for-service patients. At this time, there
is not much capitation activity, but management is
concerned that the organization must develop the
ability to manage capitated lives to prepare for the
anticipated market shifts. Community's medical staff
is composed of solo practitioners and small single-
specialty groups. The plan for medical staff development has identified a need for 30 to 40 new primary
care physicians. Virtually all of the hospital's medical
staff members are doing well financially, but all are
acutely aware of the pressures from third-party payers to reduce utilization and fees.

Nearby Major Medical Group stands out as a practice with much potential for growth. The group built a
new facility six years ago and, since that time, has
tripled in size to 21 primary care physicians. It owns
three strategically located satellite sites, and it would
like to expand further. The physicians are reasonably
productive and, due to a favorable payer mix and a
well-run business office, they are well compensated.
Although there seems to be additional opportunity for
growth in the fee-for-service part of the market, the
group leaders believe that it is time for the group to
develop some capitation experience. At the same time,
the leadership is concerned that it simply does not
have the critical mass to take substantial business risk.
Past growth has left Major Medical burdened with
significant facility-related debt, and consequently the
capital requirements associated with future expansion
are a matter of serious concern. In addition, the group
is concerned with the management challenges associ-

ated with this growth. Finally, it is uneasy about declining reimbursements and is anxious to control overhead expenses.

Both the medical group and the hospital are sensitive to the local political environment, and each is uncomfortable with a potential situation in which Major Medical Group would triple in size to meet Community's targeted development of primary care medical staff. It is clear, however, that Major Medical Group can be an important element in the hospital's overall development scheme. As a result, the two parties agree to evaluate a transaction for formation of a hospital-owned Management Service Organization (MSO) with Major Medical Group being the MSO's first client.

Baseline Financial Analysis

The development effort begins with an exploration of the financial dynamics of the Major Medical Group under a baseline scenario. The key assumptions underlying that analysis are:

1. A fixed number of physicians and productivity.

2. Constant payer mix as follows:

Commercial	30.3%
Medicare	35.5
Blue Cross	19.2
Medicaid	5.0
Other discounted	10.0
Total	100.0%

3. Collection rate changes as follows:

	1993	**1998**
Commercial	100%	100%
Medicare	85%	66%
Blue Cross	84%	80%
Medicaid	60%	40%
Other discounted	90%	86%

The results of this analysis are sobering. Compensation of the 15 partners of Major Medical Group is based on salary plus bonus. To maintain the 1998 bonus pool at 1993 levels, gross price increases need to exceed cost increases by 1.5 percent per year. Failure to maintain a differential will wipe out the bonus pool by 1998, resulting in a large decline in partner compensation. On the other hand, a pricing policy that is too aggressive will certainly put pressure on the group's base of commercially insured patients and may result in loss of those patients.

The modest conversion to capitation targeted by the group's leadership does not appear to be a better solution. Replacing a portion of existing utilization with only 10,000 capitated lives at $16 per member per month, will, with all other things constant, also wipe out the bonus pool.

Business Plan

A business plan for Major Medical Group is developed over the course of several weeks of meetings between the hospital and the group's key physicians. Important elements of the plan include the following:

1. *Group growth.* Two physicians will be added each year over the next five years. It is determined that this growth can be accommodated at existing sites. Additional sites would be identified as targets of opportunity and evaluated on an incremental basis.

2. *Capital investment.* An investment of approximately $1.6 million will be necessary to accommodate the targeted physician growth and to provide appropriate upgrades to the group's computer systems to support productivity increases.

3. *Patient volume.* The hospital is very interested in the group developing a primary care capitation base. Growth to approximately 18,000 capitated lives is targeted. Responsibility for the capitated lives is to be apportioned among existing and new physicians. It is expected that new physicians would eventually generate significant fee-for-service revenue as well. The volume projections assume a 50 percent increase in visit productivity per physician. This increase is not deemed unreasonable given the business system improvements and the group's position relative to Medical Group Management Association averages, but it is clear that the character of the practice will change substantially.

4. *Nonphysician staffing.* Assuming a fixed ratio of support staff to physicians, an additional 43 FTEs are projected, many of whom are to be

housed in currently used space at the group's main site.

The results of this business planning effort are encouraging. The financial projections show that the amount of distributable cash (the bonus pool) that the plan generates has the following improvement over the baseline:

Year	Free Cash ($000s)
1994	$(100)
1995	300
1996	700
1997	1,000
1998	1,500

Transaction Definition

Leaders of both parties focus considerable time and attention on developing an appropriate operating structure for their relationship. After several rounds of negotiation, the major points of the preliminary agreement are as follows:

1. Community General Hospital will form an MSO that will provide all nonphysician and non-real estate services to Major Medical Group in exchange for a fixed percentage of collections.

2. The hospital will provide the funds necessary to fund practice development. This provision makes sense because a significant portion of this investment could be used to support other phy-

sician practices, should the MSO develop further.

Several items are worthy of note:

1. The hospital is not interested in negotiating the purchase of the facilities, since it is not particularly interested in taking real estate risk.

2. The hospital is concerned that its management percentage will not be adequate over the long run. As a result, it negotiates a "stop loss" provision, which will become active in year four and which will limit future losses.

3. Both parties agreed to defer discussion of upfront payments until it is clear that they have established a stable operating structure.

Transaction Microeconomics

The next step is to analyze the proposed revenue and expense sharing arrangement from the individual perspectives of the two entities. Table 6-1 displays some salient data.

The following inferences may be drawn from Table 6-1:

1. *Revenue sharing.* The widely used "percentage of net revenues collected" approach to sharing revenues can pose problems in an evolving environment. Total MSO expenses grow from 37.7 percent of net revenue in year one to 42.4 percent of net revenues by year five.

Table 6-1   Analysis of Revenue and Expense Sharing

	Year 1	Year 2	Year 3	Year 4	Year 5
Aggregate Revenue	$10,841	$12,281	$13,994	$15,803	$17,927
Aggregate Cash Expense	9,895	11,060	12,374	13,815	15,430
Net	954	1,229	1,628	1,997	2,506
Major Medical Group					
Net Before Stop Loss	1,179	1,686	2,332	3,005	3,843
Stop Loss Payment	—	—	—	(208)	(1,337)
Net	1,179	1,686	2,332	2,797	2,506
Cumulative Gain	1,179	2,865	5,187	7,984	10,490
Community MSO					
Net Before Stop Loss	(226)	(458)	(704)	(1,008)	(1,337)
Stop Loss Payment	—	—	—	208	1,337
Net	(226)	(458)	(704)	(800)	0
Cumulative Loss	$(226)	$(684)	$(1,338)	$(2,188)	$(2,188)

2. *Stability*. It is apparent that the transaction is unstable from the point of view of the MSO. Break-even operation in year five is attained through a significant stop loss payment. A payment of this size probably will not sit well with the physician group either, since it will reduce compensation between years four and five.

3. *Fairness*. Obviously, there is no allowance for a return on the hospital's investment given this business plan and operating arrangement.

As a further test of what is driving the transaction's economics, a sensitivity analysis is developed in which the projected capitation volume is converted to fee-for-service volume at the payer mix and reimbursement rates included in the baseline. The results of that analysis are displayed in Table 6-2.

Although the results of the analysis are a little on the extreme side, they help to highlight two additional points:

1. This structure provides almost no upside potential to the MSO.

2. The medical group has a significant financial incentive to discourage capitation.

These and the previously described considerations lead to the conclusion that the business plan and transaction structure need revision.

Table 6-2   Fee for Service Sensitivity Analysis

	Year 1	Year 2	Year 3	Year 4	Year 5
Aggregate Revenue	$10,910	$13,279	$16,318	$19,858	$24,196
Aggregate Cash Expense	9,895	11,060	12,374	13,815	15,430
Net Income	1,015	2,219	3,944	6,043	8,766
Major Medical Group					
Net Income	1,244	2,373	3,904	5,729	8,038
Community MSO					
Net Income	(229)	(154)	40	314	728

Transaction Revision

The focus of transaction revision efforts is first trained on the business plan. After some reflection, the physicians opt for a more conservative assumption as to practice growth; the number of new physicians planned is reduced from 10 to six. The targeted number of capitated lives is reduced by 2,000, and physician productivity is not projected to increase significantly. The impact of the changes is to reduce aggregate 1998 revenues by $3.3 million. With the reduced level in visits per physician, it is determined that the number of nonphysician FTEs per physician can be decreased from 4.3 to 3.7; this contributes to a substantial reduction in operating expenses from the previous business plan. Capital expenditures are not expected to change greatly under the new plan.

A significant source of the problem is that the percentage of collection allocated to the MSO was based on the current economic model of practice, which is being fundamentally altered by growth and capitation activities. As currently structured, the MSO's share is meant to cover costs which are primarily volume driven, while the Medical Group residual was associated with significant fixed cost components. Hence the divergence in operating performance between the MSO and the group as volume grows.

One lever for problem solving involves the reconfiguration of the real estate relationship. Although both parties agree that the physicians shouldn't necessarily receive an increasing payment to cover a fixed obligation, the physicians are reluctant to accept risk for a fixed real estate payment since the MSO's decisions could potentially affect the funds available to make loan payments. To respond to this, hospital management agrees that the MSO will lease the real estate from the physicians who own it and will provide all real estate and medical equipment to Major Medical Group as part of its management fee. Community General Hospital agrees to guarantee the lease payment by the MSO.

Although this proposal has the effect of reducing the physician's percentage revenue split, it produces a tangible financial benefit. Interest rates have dropped since the facilities were financed originally. With lease payments guaranteed by the hospital, the lender is willing to loan at a reduced rate without personal guarantees by the physicians. The lower rate coupled with the fixed loan payment allow for a larger building loan, which in turn provides cash for a tax free distribution to the building's owners.

On further discussion, the hospital agrees to guarantee that partner compensation will not fall below a percentage of current compensation. Review of the revised business plan indicates that this can be achieved by allocating a fixed share of collections to the original partners.

The result of the above-described revisions is a stable transaction with more evenly distributed economic consequences, as shown in Table 6-3.

Table 6-3   Result of Revised Transaction

	Year 1	Year 2	Year 3	Year 4	Year 5
Prior MSO Income	(226)	(458)	(704)	(800)	0
Revised MSO Income	$1,412	$1,532	$1,632	$1,485	$1,296

In this revised scheme, partner compensation increases by more than 25 percent during the planning period, the pressure for volume is less intense, and some capitation experience is being developed. The partners make less money, but they have reduced operating risk, reduced personal debt loads, and an increased compensation from the baseline. In addition, they recognize that moving additional income to the MSO will enable them to generate additional benefits in the valuation process.

Valuation

The last set of analyses and negotiations has to do with upfront payments to Major Medical Group. As is the case in many markets, the group has several options available. A key consideration for each potential suitor is the potential inpatient utilization associated with the transaction. Fortunately for Community General Hospital, it is illegal to base payments on these considerations. The valuation approach with which the hospital's lawyer and auditor are most comfortable applies strict corporate finance principles to the direct economics of the transaction at hand.

The business planning and transaction development approach make this valuation straightforward. Free cash flows are estimated, and net present value assuming a middle-of-the-road 17 percent discount rate is calculated, as in Table 6-4.

Based on the advice of counsel, the hospital feels comfortable in providing and the physicians feel com-

Table 6-4   Free Cash Flows and Net Present Value

Year	Net Cash Income	Working Capital Increase	Capital Expend- itures	Free Cash	Present Value
1	$1,412	$(123)	$(320)	$969	$828
2	1,532	(102)	(320)	1,110	810
3	1,632	(108)	(320)	1,204	751
4	1,485	(27)	(320)	1,138	607
5	1,296	(20)	(320)	956	436
Terminal Value				5,623	2,564
Total					**$5,996**

fortable in accepting an offer in the range of $6 million.

Conclusion

The success that your healthcare organization will enjoy in its physician integration efforts has probably been defined already. Unless you can convince the physicians in question that your organization is going to be a player over the long run, you won't be seen as an attractive partner. This requires that you systematically apply the principles described in this book. At the same time, the care with which you approach these transactions will say a lot about the quality of management in place at your organization. Whereas others may follow the "deal a day" imperative, it is our belief that quality physicians will gravitate toward quality management; it is the well-managed and financially capable healthcare organizations that will ultimately prevail.

Afterword

Kenneth Kaufman

Quantitative Reasoning and the Financially Competitive Healthcare Organization

In this book we have tried to frame and answer two important questions:

1. Which concepts and executive skills translate into first-class financial leadership?

2. What is the balance between organizational process and analytic technique that leads to capable financial management?

What these questions suggest is that careful and rational decisionmaking in today's complex healthcare environment is difficult. The importance of financial skills and competent analysis in meeting such difficulties is obvious to observers and executives alike. Yet the need to reason quantitatively, to create an analytic context for financial decisionmaking, is given greater weight by the types of problems and organizational tendencies that interfere with executive competence.

Thomas Gilovich recently wrote a book titled *How We Know What Isn't So—The Fallibility of Human Reason in Everyday Life* [New York: The Free Press, 1991.] In this book, Professor Gilovich describes a series of observed behaviors (supported by research) that cause individuals to reason to incorrect or inappropriate conclusions. Although the author's research is addressed toward the reasoning of individuals, many of his conclusions are also appropriate to organizations. Some of the problems he has identified are addressed below:

1. *Messy data and unclear information.* Gilovich notes that the world (and, we might note, especially the healthcare world) does not play fair. Organizations are provided not with clear information but instead with a data set that Gilovich characterizes as random, incomplete, nonrepresentative, ambiguous, inconsistent, and generally secondhand. Gilovich notes that the attempts to cope with a messy data set often reveal inferential shortcomings, which lead to wrong conclusions. One example of messy data and unclear information is the current attempt by many healthcare organizations to project the financial results of short hospitalizations. As a result of pressure from third-party payers to eliminate all

but the most necessary admissions, many hospitals now admit patients for less than a day for diagnostic and treatment services. The data on reimbursement and costs for such brief admissions are in some cases unavailable and in other cases incomplete and ambiguous. Attempts to properly project revenue and resource consumption in environments with increasing short hospital stays is extremely difficult. The analytic obstacles are significant, but the example is quite clear. An organization's ability to reason its way around and through a messy data set of this type is a critical prerequisite to capable financial decisionmaking.

2. *Pattern phenomena.* As Gilovich points out, individuals and organizations tend to detect patterns and order phenomena where no such order exists. His fascinating example for pattern phenomena is the concept of streak shooting in basketball. Players, coaches, and fans alike are convinced that the notion of streak shooting ("the hot hand," "in the zone"), in fact, exists. As a result, coaches and players make decisions, which often affect the outcomes of games, based on the supposed existence of streak shooting.

The problem is that the notion of streak shooting cannot be statistically validated. Gilovich's research of shooting statistics for professional basketball teams demonstrated that the pattern of shots made and missed always falls within statistically expected margins. In other words, the shooting performance of any player at any given time is not predictable, it is statistically random. As Gilovich points out, individuals believe firmly in "pattern and order" and make decisions accordingly.

An example of pattern phenomena in healthcare might include the relationship of utilization and intensity of care to resource consumption. Healthcare executives may operate on the assumption that certain levels of specific utilization will lead directly to certain levels of resource requirements. Many executives make strategic and financial decisions based on the assumption of order in these relationships. Yet it is possible that these relationships are not ordered but subject to significant variability depending on management attitudes, physician decision-making, and pressure from managed care organizations and third-party payers.

In how many other situations in healthcare organizations do we see order and pattern where no order and pattern exists? Which types of decisions do we make on the basis of these patterns? And most importantly, which types of analyses are necessary to properly identify and categorize information in a way that permits executives to reason to correct and supportable outcomes?

3. *Overemphasis of positive data.* Gilovich says, "People are inclined to see what they expect to see, and conclude what they expect to conclude. Information that is consistent with . . . preexisting beliefs is often accepted at face value, whereas

evidence that contradicts them is critically discounted."

There is almost a natural tendency to over-value data that confirm preexisting beliefs; coping with the inevitable overemphasis of positive data requires hard-edge analysis. A reliance on so-called soft management skills (intuition) exacerbates the tendency to support favored hypotheses without giving possible alternatives a fair evaluation.

The most vivid example of this tendency in healthcare is in the acquisition process. It is our experience that many management teams make the acquisition decision first and complete the analysis last. It is our further observation that the slightest positive data will serve to confirm an already-made purchase decision, whereas no amount of opposing data and conflicting analysis can slow the buy decision.

4. *The Lake Wobegon effect.* Garrison Keillor says that in his fictional setting Lake Wobegon, "the women are strong, the men are good looking, and all the children are above average." Psychologists call this inclination to adopt self-serving and comfortable beliefs about the world the Lake Wobegon effect.

Many observers have noted that acute care delivered in capital-intensive environments is a phenomenon of the past. Yet J. Ian Morrison has commented, "What killed the railways was that they were run by people who really liked choo-choos. This is also the Achilles' heel of hospitals.

They are run by people fascinated with big white buildings and all they contain." ("Railways of the Nineties," Healthcare Forum Journal, March, April, 1994.)

On the contrary, we believe that most healthcare executives are not fascinated by buildings and technology; they are simply "comforted" by the Lake Wobegon effect, in this case by capital-intensive practices and beliefs that have been successful in the past. Such comforting practices are extremely difficult to abandon and if held too long, lead to major investment decisions and strategic decisions whose value is past.

5. *Ambiguous criteria.* Individuals and organizations reason for results. Gilovich points out that decisions which lead to successful outcomes naturally stimulate similar decisions. Furthermore, the more ambiguous the criterion used, the easier it is to detect evidence of success. For-profit corporations have clear definitions of success—if profits increase or the stock price increases, the evaluative criteria have been met. Evaluative criteria in the not-for-profit sector are messy. Criteria for success can include financial goals, mission goals, or standards of community health. This is problematic in that Gilovich notes, "The more ambiguous the criteria, the easier it is to declare yourself successful and the easier it is to repeat decisions which may, in fact, be misdirected and wrong headed."

The critical problems of organizational decision-making set out above cannot be overcome by hard work alone. Financial competence requires real skills, appropriate attitudes, sustained leadership, and a consistent decisionmaking process, all, in turn, supported by an expert analytic technique.

Leadership is provided by a senior management that is willing to identify an appropriate financial vision for the organization and communicate that vision to essential constituencies. Another requirement is a financial planning process that provides a critical framework for acquiring the necessary financial resources to implement the desired strategy and any investment analysis needed to support such a strategy.

This line of thought leads to a final critical distinction relative to the development of capable financial leadership: there is a meaningful difference between the competent preparation of analyses and the consumption, or use, of those same analyses. The chart in Figure 7-1 is instructive of this distinction.

Figure 7-1 Organizational Analysis and Decisionmaking

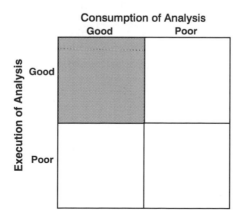

To reason through and around the problems posed by Gilovich, an organization must commit to the use of the scientific method and the quantitative analyses that support the creation and testing of alternate hypotheses. Most organizations believe that they have fulfilled this requirement by creating analytic rigor at the appropriate level of the executive team. But as the chart demonstrates, the capable healthcare organization recognizes that financial management requires not only creative and competent analysis but also the receptive consumption of that analysis. The ability to solve financial problems and make consistent and excellent investment decisions is accomplished only within the shaded quadrant of the chart. Recognize that only a few managers prepare the analyses on which organizational decisions are made. The majority of executives are the consumers and use such analyses to make decisions. The process cannot serve the organization well if the executive team is not prepared in both attitude and training to appropriately use the analytic tools and techniques provided.

It is important to remember that healthcare is not just another business. Healthcare involves the delivery of care and resources to people, many of whom are in their time of greatest need. Yet from a more pragmatic perspective healthcare is a business. This is true because healthcare organizations, like commercial enterprises, must accurately estimate resource requirements and then operate at levels which meet both short and long term financial needs. Human and financial capital must be raised and growth must be accomodated. All of this must be accomplished through a decisionmaking process that continuously copes with seemingly insolvable problems and contradictory alternatives. The principles and methods set out in this book provide an essential foundation to assist healthcare organizations in reasoning through the complex issues that confront the industry today. The principles of finance and analysis are not a substitute for executive experience and judgment. These principles, however, do provide a critical analytic framework that when combined with judgment and experience will permit healthcare organizations to remain financially competitive and meet the challenges of a demanding and uncertain marketplace.

Index

Integration analysis,
    see Physician-hospital
Interest, 63
  see Capitalized
Interest rate, 35, 56, 61, 141,
    172
  see Market
  assumptions, 35
Internal benchmarking
    process, 12
Intuition, 3
Inventory, 59
  see Capital
Investment
  see Risk-free, Upfront
  amount, 123
  analysis, 49, 50-68, 128
    case study, 67-68
    goals, 49, 50-51
    theory, 49
    theory/process, 51-67
  banker, 89
  decision, 48, 49, 54
    financing decision,
      separation, 97
  opportunities, 7, 39
  scenario, 72, 73

L
Lake Wobegon effect, 179-180
Leadership, 181
  team, 95, 99
Leverage, 130
  ratio, 32, 89
Liquidation
  approach, 75
  value, 65
Liquidity, 22, 30
  ratio, 32

  requirements, 11
Long-term
  capital constraints, 77
  capital investment, 29
  capital plan, 125
  capital requirements, 16, 20
    definition, 20-28
    questions, 20-24
  competitive position, 20
  debt borrowing rate, 99
  financial
    competitiveness, 123
    goals, 32, 123
    performance, 6
    plan, 125
    requirements, 18, 24
    success, 13
    targets, 32, 123
  organizational financial
    goals, 124
  profitability targets, 21, 23
  strategy, 27
  success, 48
  value, 9

M
Macroeconomics,
    see Transaction
Major Medical Group, 162,
    164, 166
Managed care, 69
  contracts, 101, 105
  environment, 68
  issues, 149
  products, 150
  strategy, 2
  utilization, 72
  volume, 105
Management, 6-11, 109, 157

investment, 58
Utilization, 27, 102, 103, 108,
    110, 120, 154
  see Medicare
  data, 102
  growth variables, 102-103
  information, 102
Utilization-by-payer data, 111

V
Valuation analysis, 111-114
Value
  see Long-term
  estimate, *see* Terminal
Visibility of consequences, 11
Volatility, *see* Financial
    performance
Volume, 54, 142

  see Patient
Vulnerability, 134
  key variables, 102

W
Weighting structures, 84
What-if
  analysis, 55
  scenarios, 42
Working capital, 17, 101
  needs, *see* Incremental
  requirements, 59, 72

Y
Year-to-date financial
  performance, 116
  statement, 102

About the Authors

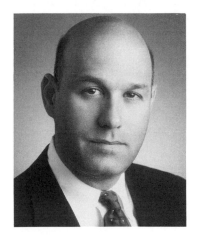

Kenneth Kaufman, Managing Director

Mr. Kaufman is a founder and Managing Director of Kaufman, Hall & Associates. His experience encompasses virtually all areas of capital advisory services.

Since 1976, Mr. Kaufman has consulted to healthcare organizations throughout the country in capital planning, joint venture development, financial advisory services and mergers and acquisitions. He has also developed a particular expertise in governance evaluation and organization.

Mr. Kaufman is an important contributor to the healthcare field. During the past five years, he has presented over one hundred programs to audiences throughout the United States including seminars sponsored by the ACHE, the AHA, the HFMA, the AGPA and the MGMA.

Mr. Kaufman is the co-author of *The Capital Management of Health Care Organizations*. In addition, his articles have appeared in most major healthcare publications including *Healthcare Financial Management, Trustee, Modern Healthcare* and *Hospitals*. Mr. Kaufman holds a Masters Degree in Business Administration from the University of Chicago Graduate School of Business with a concentration in hospital administration.

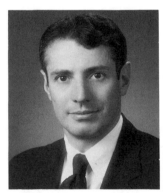

Mark Hall, Director

A founder and Director of Kaufman, Hall & Associates, Mr. Hall has served as financial advisor to a wide range of healthcare organizations throughout the United States since 1977.

Prior to founding KHA, Mr. Hall was a Senior Vice President for a major midwest financial consulting firm. In addition, Mr. Hall was a consultant in A.T.

Kearney's healthcare practice where he specialized in strategic planning and financial analysis.

Mr. Hall has extensive experience in capital planning, financial advisory services, mergers and acquisitions, as well as organizing and reorganizing joint venture and diversification activities. He is particularly interested in the application of corporate finance principles to management of nonprofit organizations.

Mr. Hall is a regular contributor to the healthcare field. His activities have included numerous articles and speaking engagements for such organizations as the AHA, the HFMA and the ACHE. He is the co-author of *The Capital Management of Health Care Organizations*.

Mr. Hall holds a Masters Degree in Business Administration from the University of Chicago Graduate School of Business with a concentration in Hospital Administration and a Bachelors Degree in Economics from Amherst College.